GASTRIC ULCER DIET COOKBOOK FOR BEGINNERS

Quick and Nutritious Anti-Inflammatory Recipes to Alleviate Ulcer Symptoms and Promote Digestive Health

Kingsley Klopp

To show our appreciation for your purchase, we're delighted to offer you these special bonuses as a heartfelt thank you.

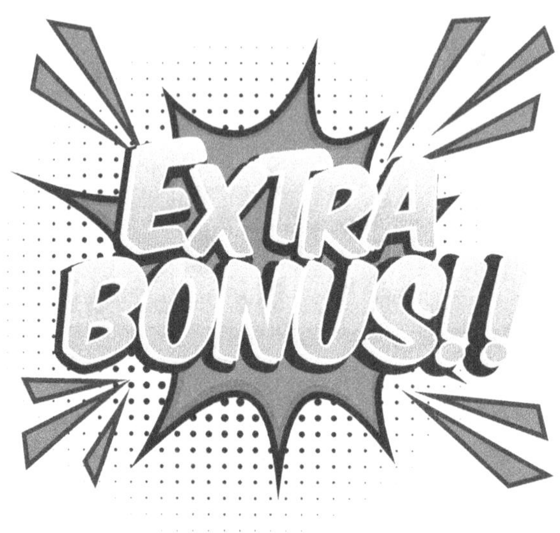

1. A Food Tracker Journal
2. Downloadable E-BOOK featuring full-color images of finished recipes

Table of Contents

Poultry Recipes

Important Note

Before you dive into these pages filled with delicious and healing recipes, we want to emphasize a few important points. Everyone's body is unique, and individual dietary needs can vary significantly. While the recipes in this cookbook are designed with sensitivity to gastric ulcers in mind, it's essential to listen to your body and make adjustments as necessary to suit your personal needs and preferences.

Consulting with your healthcare provider or a registered dietitian is strongly advised, especially if you have any uncertainties or specific health concerns regarding your diet. They can provide personalized guidance and ensure that the dietary choices you make align with your overall treatment plan and health goals.

Please also note that the nutritional information provided with each recipe is approximate. Variations in ingredient brands, portion sizes, and preparation methods can impact the final nutritional content of your meals. Use this information as a general guideline and consider it alongside professional advice for a comprehensive understanding of your dietary intake.

As you explore the recipes within this cookbook, we encourage you to approach them with curiosity and creativity. Discover new flavors, adapt recipes to suit your preferences, and enjoy the process of nourishing yourself with meals that support your digestive health and overall well-being.

Furthermore, If our cookbook has brought joy to your kitchen and table, we'd be thrilled to hear about your experiences in an Amazon review. On the flip side, if you stumble upon any hiccups while exploring our recipes, don't hesitate to get in touch at **kloppkingsley@gmail.com.** We're here to support your cooking journey every step of the way.

We understand that managing gastric ulcers can be challenging, but remember that you are not alone on this journey. Together, let's embrace the healing power of food and empower ourselves with knowledge and delicious recipes that make everyday meals a source of comfort and support.

Introduction

Imagine waking up each morning with a persistent ache in your stomach, a reminder that every meal comes with its own set of challenges. Living with a gastric ulcer isn't just about what you eat—it's about finding a way to nourish your body while soothing the discomfort that accompanies every bite. That's where the **Gastric Ulcer Diet Cookbook for Beginners** comes in, offering you a pathway to delicious, healing meals that support your journey to better digestive health.

Let's face it: dealing with a gastric ulcer can be overwhelming. The pain, the burning sensation, the uncertainty about what foods will trigger symptoms—all of these can make mealtime a dreaded affair. But it doesn't have to be that way. This cookbook is your guide to navigating the culinary landscape with confidence and creativity, ensuring that every meal you prepare not only satisfies your taste buds but also nurtures your stomach. Cooking for a gastric ulcer requires a delicate balance of flavors and nutrients. You want meals that are gentle on your stomach yet satisfying enough to keep you energized throughout the day. Our cookbook is packed with easy-to-follow recipes that prioritize ingredients known for their soothing properties, helping to calm inflammation and promote healing. From comforting broths and soothing herbal teas to hearty yet gentle main courses, each recipe is crafted with your digestive well-being in mind. But this cookbook isn't just about recipes. It's about empowering you with the knowledge and confidence to take charge of your diet and health. We provide practical tips on ingredient selection, meal planning, and portion control, ensuring that you have the tools to create balanced, ulcer-friendly meals at home. Understanding your condition is key to managing it effectively, and we're here to support you every step of the way.

One of the biggest challenges of living with a gastric ulcer is the uncertainty surrounding what to eat. Foods that once brought pleasure may now cause discomfort, leaving you feeling frustrated and deprived. Our goal is to show you that eating for health can still be enjoyable. Through innovative recipes and creative adaptations, we'll help you rediscover the joy of cooking and eating, one delicious dish at a time. We understand that everyone's experience with gastric ulcers is unique. What works for one person may not work for another, and that's okay. Our cookbook encourages you to experiment with different flavors and ingredients, allowing you to tailor each recipe to suit your individual preferences and dietary needs. Whether you're a seasoned chef or a kitchen novice, you'll find inspiration and encouragement within these pages to create meals that nourish both body and soul.

In addition to recipes, we provide insights into lifestyle adjustments that can complement your dietary choices. From stress management techniques to the importance of hydration and regular exercise, holistic well-being is at the heart of our approach. Eating well is just one piece of the puzzle; taking care of your overall health is essential for managing gastric ulcers effectively.

As you set out on this culinary journey with us, remember that healing takes time and patience. There will be ups and downs, good days and challenging days. But through it all, know that you're not alone. The "**Gastric Ulcer Diet Cookbook for Beginner**s is here to support you, offering delicious recipes, practical advice, and a sense of community as you work towards better digestive health. So, gather your ingredients, sharpen your knives, and let's cook our way to wellness together. With each meal you prepare, you're taking a positive step towards healing and embracing a lifestyle that supports your health and happiness.

Part 1: Understanding Gastric Ulcers

What is a Gastric Ulcer?

A gastric ulcer, often referred to as a peptic ulcer, is a painful open sore that forms on the lining of the stomach. It's a condition that has affected countless lives, causing immense discomfort and distress. But to truly understand what a gastric ulcer is, we need to delve into its history, its development, and the profound impact it has had on humanity.

The Historical Journey of Gastric Ulcers

The story of gastric ulcers is as old as human civilization itself. Ancient medical texts from Egypt, Greece, and China contain references to stomach pain and digestive issues that we now recognize as symptoms of ulcers. The Greek physician Hippocrates, often called the father of medicine, described conditions that closely resemble modern-day gastric ulcers. Despite this early recognition, the true nature of these painful sores remained a mystery for millennia. In the 19th century, advancements in medical science began to shed light on gastric ulcers. With the invention of the endoscope, doctors could finally see inside the human stomach, and the sight was often shocking: red, inflamed sores marring the delicate lining of the stomach. These visual revelations brought a new urgency to understand and treat this debilitating condition.

The Nature of Gastric Ulcers

At its core, a gastric ulcer is a breach in the protective mucous lining of the stomach. This lining serves as a barrier against the harsh acidic environment necessary for digestion. When this barrier is compromised, stomach acid can erode the stomach's tissue, leading to the formation of an ulcer. The pain of a gastric ulcer is not just physical; it can be deeply emotional as well. Imagine the sharp, burning sensation in your stomach, often striking unexpectedly and leaving you clutching your abdomen in agony. This pain can disrupt daily life, making simple activities like eating and sleeping a challenge. For many, it can feel like a constant battle against an unseen enemy.

Evolution of Understanding and Treatment

The understanding of gastric ulcers has evolved dramatically over the years. Initially, it was believed that stress and spicy foods were the primary culprits. This led to treatments focused on lifestyle changes and bland diets, which offered limited relief to sufferers.

A groundbreaking moment in the history of gastric ulcers came in the 1980s, when Australian scientists Barry Marshall and Robin Warren discovered that a bacterium called Helicobacter pylori (H. pylori) was a major cause of many ulcers. This discovery revolutionized the medical community's approach to ulcers. No longer were they seen merely as a consequence of stress or diet; they were now understood as a condition that could be treated with antibiotics. Marshall and Warren's discovery was initially met with skepticism. To prove their point, Marshall famously ingested a solution containing H. pylori, subsequently developing gastritis, which he then treated successfully with antibiotics. This daring experiment not only won them a Nobel Prize but also paved the way for millions of ulcer sufferers to find relief.

Living with a gastric ulcer is a journey marked by highs and lows. The physical pain is often accompanied by a profound emotional toll. The fear of eating something that might trigger an episode, the anxiety of living with chronic pain, and the frustration of recurring symptoms can be overwhelming. Many people find themselves feeling isolated, unable to enjoy meals with family and friends, and struggling to maintain a sense of normalcy. But amidst the struggle, there is hope. The medical advancements in understanding and treating gastric ulcers have transformed what was once a life-altering condition into a manageable one. Modern treatments, including antibiotics for H. pylori and proton pump inhibitors to reduce stomach acid, have given many their lives back.

For anyone who has suffered from a gastric ulcer, the journey is deeply personal. It's a testament to human resilience and the relentless pursuit of relief and healing. The scars left by an ulcer are not just physical; they are also emotional, reminding us of the battles we've fought and the strength we've discovered within ourselves. A gastric ulcer is much more than a medical condition. It is a story of human perseverance, scientific discovery, and the enduring hope for a pain-free life. As we continue to learn and grow, both individually and as a society, the fight against gastric ulcers reminds us of the incredible progress we've made and the brighter future that lies ahead for all who suffer from this challenging condition.

Causes and Symptoms of Gastric Ulcers

Causes of Gastric Ulcers
1. Helicobacter pylori (H. pylori) Infection: One of the most common causes of gastric ulcers is an infection with the bacterium Helicobacter pylori. This bacterium disrupts the protective mucous layer of the stomach, making it more susceptible to damage from stomach acid. The discovery of H. pylori as a major cause of ulcers revolutionized our understanding and treatment of the condition. H. pylori is typically contracted through contaminated food or water and can persist for years, causing chronic inflammation and ulceration if not treated.
2. Nonsteroidal Anti-Inflammatory Drugs (NSAIDs): Regular use of NSAIDs, such as aspirin, ibuprofen, and naproxen, is another significant cause of gastric ulcers. These medications inhibit the production of certain chemicals that protect the stomach lining, increasing the risk of ulcer formation. Prolonged use or high doses of NSAIDs can cause significant irritation and erosion of the stomach lining, leading to ulcers.
3. Excess Stomach Acid Production: Conditions that increase stomach acid production, such as Zollinger-Ellison syndrome, can also lead to the development of gastric ulcers. Excess acid can overwhelm the stomach's protective mechanisms, leading to ulceration. Stress, while not a direct cause, can exacerbate this condition by increasing acid production.
4. Smoking and Alcohol Consumption: Smoking cigarettes and consuming alcohol can also contribute to the development of gastric ulcers. Smoking increases stomach acid and reduces the production of bicarbonate, a substance that helps neutralize stomach acid. Alcohol, particularly when consumed in large quantities, can irritate and erode the stomach lining, making it more susceptible to ulcer formation.
5. Dietary Factors: While diet alone is not typically a primary cause of gastric ulcers, certain foods and beverages can exacerbate the condition. Spicy foods, caffeine, and acidic foods like citrus fruits can irritate the stomach lining and exacerbate symptoms in people who already have ulcers.
6. Genetic Predisposition: Some individuals may be genetically predisposed to developing gastric ulcers. A family history of ulcers can increase one's risk, suggesting that genetic factors may play a role in the condition's development.

Symptoms of Gastric Ulcers

1. Abdominal Pain: The most common and prominent symptom of a gastric ulcer is a burning or gnawing pain in the abdomen, typically in the upper middle part of the stomach. This pain may be more pronounced when the stomach is empty and can often be temporarily relieved by eating certain foods that buffer stomach acid or by taking antacids.
2. Bloating and Belching: Many individuals with gastric ulcers experience frequent bloating and belching. This can be accompanied by a feeling of fullness, even after eating small amounts of food.
3. Nausea and Vomiting: Nausea, sometimes accompanied by vomiting, is another common symptom. In severe cases, vomiting may include blood, indicating bleeding from the ulcer site, which requires immediate medical attention.
4. Loss of Appetite and Weight Loss: Gastric ulcers can lead to a significant loss of appetite and unintentional weight loss. The pain and discomfort associated with eating can make food seem unappealing, leading to decreased caloric intake.
5. Heartburn and Acid Reflux: Many people with gastric ulcers experience heartburn and acid reflux. This is due to the increased acidity in the stomach and the irritation of the esophagus.
6. Dark or Tarry Stools: Ulcers can cause bleeding, which may be visible in the stool. Dark, tarry stools are a sign of gastrointestinal bleeding and should be addressed by a healthcare provider immediately.
7. Fatigue: Chronic blood loss from an ulcer can lead to anemia, causing fatigue, weakness, and pale skin. This symptom is often overlooked but is a significant indicator of an underlying problem.

The Role of Diet in Managing Gastric Ulcers

The stomach lining is protected by a mucous layer that acts as a barrier against stomach acid. When this barrier is compromised, as in the case of a gastric ulcer, the stomach lining is left vulnerable to acid erosion, leading to pain and discomfort. A proper diet can help reinforce this mucous layer, reduce acid production, and provide nutrients essential for healing.

Foods to Include in a Gastric Ulcer Diet
1. High-Fiber Foods:
   - Benefits: High-fiber foods can help reduce stomach acid levels and promote regular bowel movements, which are beneficial for overall digestive health.
   - Examples: Oatmeal, whole grains, brown rice, barley, and vegetables such as carrots, broccoli, and sweet potatoes.
2. Lean Proteins:
   - Benefits: Protein is essential for tissue repair and recovery. Lean proteins are less likely to cause excessive acid production compared to fatty meats.
   - Examples: Skinless poultry, lean beef, fish, tofu, and legumes.
3. Non-Citrus Fruits:
   - Benefits: Fruits that are low in acid can provide essential vitamins and antioxidants without irritating the stomach lining.
   - Examples: Bananas, apples, pears, melons, and berries.
4. Vegetables:
   - Benefits: Most vegetables are low in fat and sugar, making them gentle on the stomach. They also provide essential vitamins and minerals.
   - Examples: Leafy greens, carrots, zucchini, and bell peppers.
5. Fermented Foods:
   - Benefits: Fermented foods contain probiotics, which can help balance the gut microbiome and promote digestive health.
   - Examples: Yogurt, kefir, sauerkraut, and miso.
6. Healthy Fats:
   - Benefits: Healthy fats can help reduce inflammation and are easier on the stomach than saturated fats.
   - Examples: Olive oil, avocados, and nuts.
7. Whole Grains:
   - Benefits: Whole grains provide fiber, which can help regulate digestion and reduce stomach acid.
   - Examples: Whole wheat bread, brown rice, quinoa, and oats.

Foods to Avoid in a Gastric Ulcer Diet

1. Spicy Foods:
   - Risks: Spicy foods can irritate the stomach lining and exacerbate ulcer symptoms.
   - Examples: Hot peppers, chili powder, and spicy sauces.
2. Caffeinated Beverages:
   - Risks: Caffeine can increase stomach acid production and cause irritation.
   - Examples: Coffee, tea, and energy drinks.
3. Alcohol:
   - Risks: Alcohol can erode the stomach lining and increase acid production, leading to worsening symptoms.
   - Examples: Beer, wine, and spirits.
4. Acidic Foods:
   - Risks: Acidic foods can aggravate the stomach lining and increase discomfort.
   - Examples: Citrus fruits, tomatoes, and vinegar.
5. Fatty and Fried Foods:
   - Risks: High-fat foods can slow digestion and increase stomach acid, leading to irritation and discomfort.
   - Examples: Fried chicken, french fries, and fatty cuts of meat.
6. Processed Foods:
   - Risks: Processed foods often contain additives and preservatives that can irritate the stomach.
   - Examples: Packaged snacks, ready meals, and processed meats.

Meal Planning Tips for Gastric Ulcer Management

1. Eat Small, Frequent Meals:
   - Eating smaller, more frequent meals can help reduce the burden on the stomach and prevent excessive acid production. This approach can also help maintain steady energy levels throughout the day.
2. Chew Food Thoroughly:
   - Chewing food thoroughly aids in the digestive process and reduces the workload on the stomach. This can help prevent irritation and promote better nutrient absorption.
3. Avoid Eating Late at Night:
   - Eating late at night can lead to increased acid production while lying down, which can exacerbate symptoms. It's best to have your last meal a few hours before bedtime.

4. Stay Hydrated:
    - Drinking plenty of water throughout the day can help dilute stomach acid and promote digestion. However, it's important to avoid drinking large amounts of water during meals, as this can increase stomach volume and pressure.
5. Incorporate Soothing Teas:
    - Herbal teas such as chamomile, ginger, and licorice root can help soothe the stomach lining and reduce inflammation. These teas can be a comforting addition to your diet.

Breakfast Recipes

1. Oatmeal with Banana and Honey

Ingredients

- 1 cup rolled oats
- 2 cups water
- 1 cup almond milk (or any milk of your choice)
- 1 ripe banana, sliced
- 1 tablespoon honey
- 1/2 teaspoon cinnamon
- 1/4 teaspoon vanilla extract

Instructions

1. In a medium saucepan, bring the water and almond milk to a boil.
2. Add the rolled oats and reduce the heat to a simmer. Cook for about 5-7 minutes, stirring occasionally, until the oats are soft and have absorbed most of the liquid.
3. Stir in the cinnamon and vanilla extract.
4. Serve the oatmeal in bowls, topped with sliced banana and a drizzle of honey.

Nutrition Information (Per Serving)

- Calories: 220
- Protein: 5g
- Carbohydrates: 44g
- Dietary Fiber: 6g
- Sugars: 12g
- Fat: 3g
- Saturated Fat: 0g
- Cholesterol: 0mg
- Sodium: 30mg

Servings

- **2 servings**

Cooking Time

- **10 minutes**

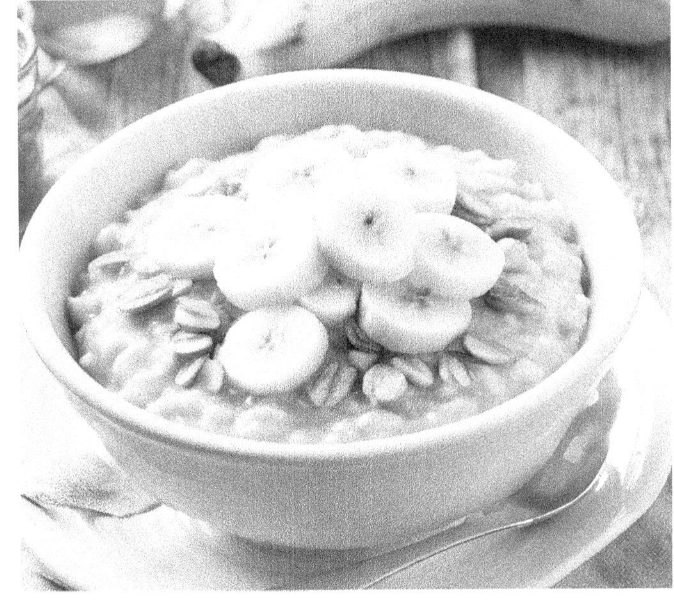

2. Creamy Rice Porridge

Ingredients

- 1 cup jasmine rice (or any white rice)
- 4 cups water
- 1 cup almond milk (or any milk of your choice)
- 1/4 teaspoon cinnamon
- 1 tablespoon honey
- 1 ripe banana, mashed
- 1/2 teaspoon vanilla extract

Instructions

1. Rinse the rice under cold water until the water runs clear.
2. In a large pot, bring the water to a boil. Add the rice and reduce the heat to a low simmer. Cook the rice for about 20 minutes or until it is very soft and begins to break down, stirring occasionally.
3. Add the almond milk, mashed banana, cinnamon, and vanilla extract. Stir well to combine.
4. Cook for an additional 10 minutes, stirring frequently, until the porridge is creamy.
5. Serve hot, drizzled with honey.

Nutrition Information (Per Serving)

- Calories: 230
- Protein: 4g
- Carbohydrates: 50g
- Dietary Fiber: 2g
- Sugars: 9g
- Fat: 2g
- Saturated Fat: 0g
- Cholesterol: 0mg
- Sodium: 25mg

Servings

- **4 servings**

Cooking Time

- **30 minutes**

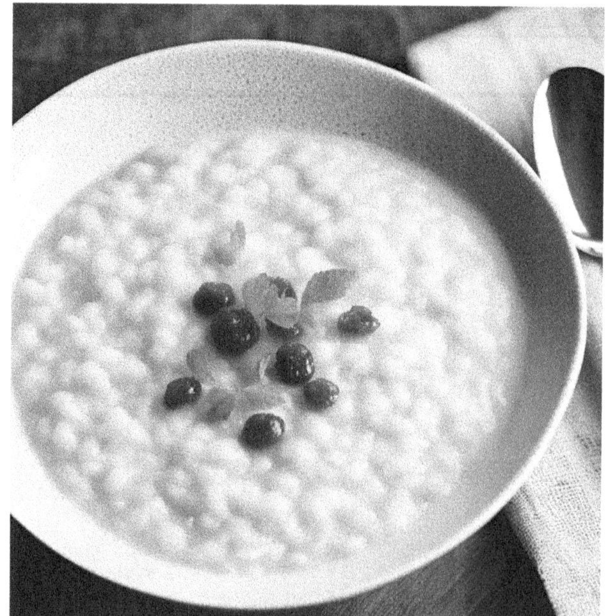

3. Avocado Toast

Ingredients

- 2 ripe avocados
- 4 slices whole grain bread
- 1/2 teaspoon olive oil
- 1/4 teaspoon ground cumin
- 1/4 teaspoon ground paprika
- 1 tablespoon lemon juice
- Freshly ground black pepper to taste

Instructions

1. Toast the whole grain bread slices until golden brown and crispy.
2. While the bread is toasting, cut the avocados in half, remove the pit, and scoop the flesh into a bowl.
3. Add the olive oil, ground cumin, ground paprika, lemon juice, and a pinch of black pepper to the avocado. Mash together with a fork until smooth and creamy.
4. Spread the mashed avocado mixture evenly onto the toasted bread slices.
5. Serve immediately.

Nutrition Information (Per Serving)

- Calories: 250
- Protein: 6g
- Carbohydrates: 28g
- Dietary Fiber: 10g
- Sugars: 2g
- Fat: 15g
- Saturated Fat: 2g
- Cholesterol: 0mg
- Sodium: 120mg

Servings

- **4 servings**

Cooking Time

- **10 minutes**

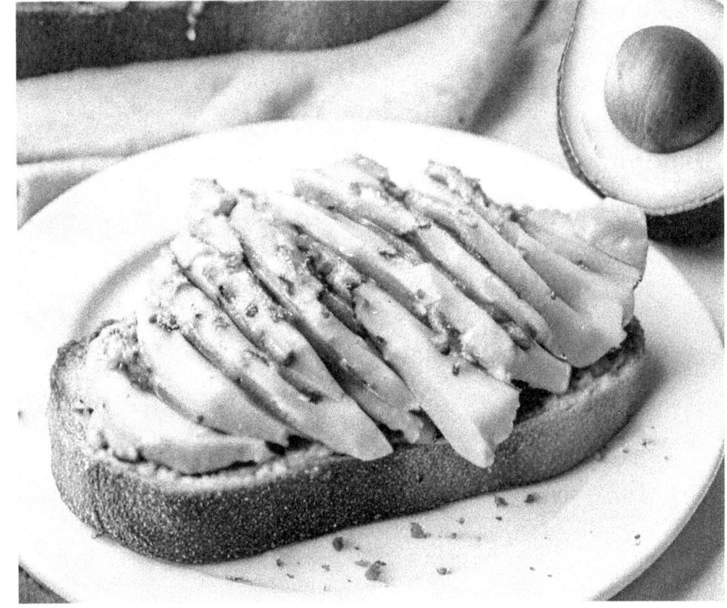

4. Cottage Cheese with Melon

Ingredients

- 2 cups cottage cheese
- 1 small cantaloupe or honeydew melon, cubed
- 1 tablespoon honey
- 1/4 teaspoon ground cinnamon
- Fresh mint leaves for garnish (optional)

Instructions

1. Cut the melon in half, remove the seeds, and scoop out the flesh into bite-sized cubes.
2. In a bowl, combine the cottage cheese and melon cubes.
3. Drizzle with honey and sprinkle with ground cinnamon.
4. Mix gently to combine.
5. Garnish with fresh mint leaves if desired and serve immediately.

Nutrition Information (Per Serving)

- Calories: 180
- Protein: 14g
- Carbohydrates: 20g
- Dietary Fiber: 2g
- Sugars: 15g
- Fat: 5g
- Saturated Fat: 3g
- Cholesterol: 20mg
- Sodium: 400mg

Servings

- **4 servings**

Cooking Time

- **10 minutes**

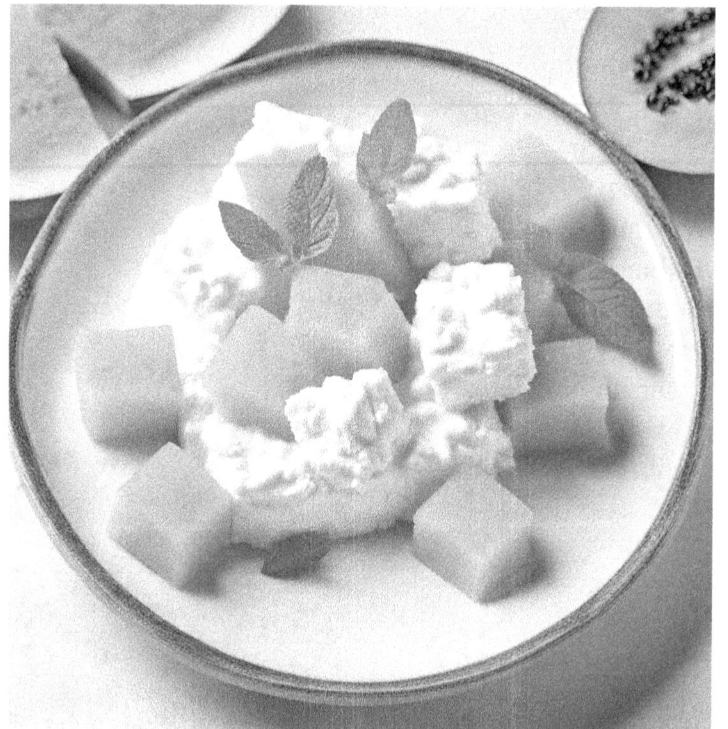

5. Steamed Sweet Potato

Ingredients

- 4 medium sweet potatoes
- 1 tablespoon olive oil
- 1/4 teaspoon ground cinnamon
- 1/4 teaspoon ground nutmeg

Instructions

1. Wash the sweet potatoes thoroughly and peel them.
2. Cut the sweet potatoes into thick slices or cubes.
3. Place the sweet potato pieces in a steamer basket over boiling water.
4. Cover and steam for about 15-20 minutes or until tender.
5. Remove the sweet potatoes from the steamer and place them in a bowl.
6. Drizzle with olive oil and sprinkle with ground cinnamon and nutmeg.
7. Toss gently to coat evenly and serve warm.

Nutrition Information (Per Serving)

- Calories: 120
- Protein: 2g
- Carbohydrates: 28g
- Dietary Fiber: 4g
- Sugars: 6g
- Fat: 3g
- Saturated Fat: 0g
- Cholesterol: 0mg
- Sodium: 40mg

Servings

- **4 servings**

Cooking Time

- **25 minutes**

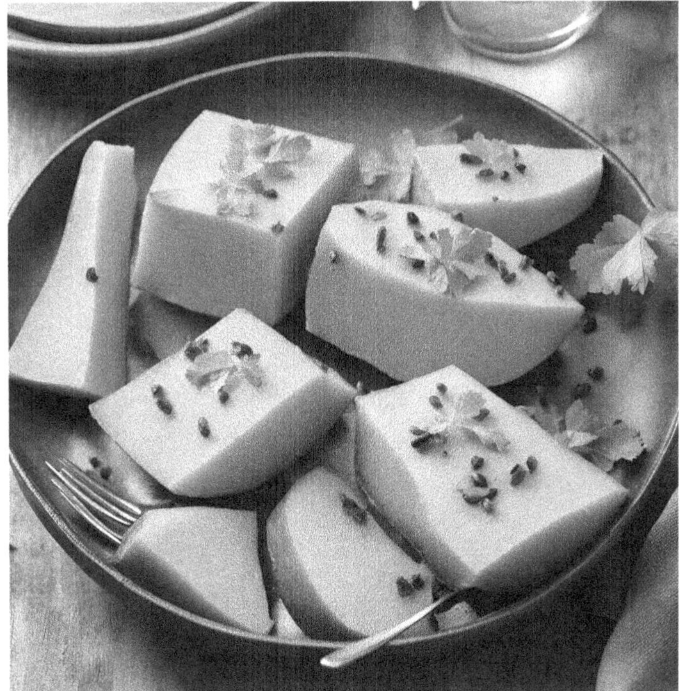

6. Applesauce Pancakes

Ingredients

- 1 cup whole wheat flour
- 1 teaspoon baking powder
- 1/2 teaspoon baking soda
- 1 teaspoon ground cinnamon
- 1/4 teaspoon ground nutmeg
- 1 cup unsweetened applesauce
- 1/2 cup almond milk (or any milk of your choice)
- 1 large egg
- 1 tablespoon honey
- 1 teaspoon vanilla extract

Instructions

1. In a large bowl, whisk together the whole wheat flour, baking powder, baking soda, ground cinnamon, and ground nutmeg.
2. In another bowl, mix the applesauce, almond milk, egg, honey, and vanilla extract until well combined.
3. Pour the wet ingredients into the dry ingredients and stir until just combined. Do not overmix.
4. Heat a non-stick skillet or griddle over medium heat.
5. Pour 1/4 cup of batter onto the skillet for each pancake.
6. Cook until bubbles form on the surface and the edges look set, about 2-3 minutes. Flip and cook for another 2-3 minutes until golden brown.
7. Serve warm with a drizzle of honey or a dollop of extra applesauce if desired.

Nutrition Information (Per Serving)

- Calories: 150
- Protein: 4g
- Carbohydrates: 28g
- Dietary Fiber: 4g
- Sugars: 10g
- Fat: 3g
- Saturated Fat: 0g
- Cholesterol: 40mg
- Sodium: 220mg

Servings

- **4 servings**

Cooking Time

- **20 minutes**

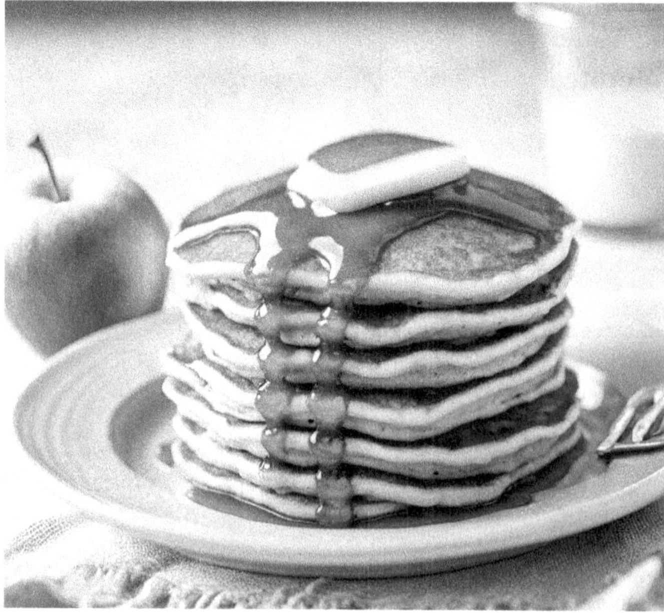

7. Pumpkin Soup

Ingredients

- 4 cups pumpkin puree (canned or fresh)
- 4 cups low-sodium vegetable broth
- 1 cup coconut milk
- 1 tablespoon olive oil
- 1/2 teaspoon ground ginger
- 1/4 teaspoon ground cinnamon
- 1/4 teaspoon ground nutmeg
- Fresh parsley for garnish (optional)

Instructions

1. In a large pot, heat the olive oil over medium heat.
2. Add the pumpkin puree, vegetable broth, coconut milk, ground ginger, ground cinnamon, and ground nutmeg.
3. Stir well to combine all ingredients.
4. Bring the mixture to a simmer and cook for about 15-20 minutes, stirring occasionally.
5. Use an immersion blender to blend the soup until smooth (or transfer to a blender in batches if you do not have an immersion blender).
6. Adjust the seasoning to taste and serve hot, garnished with fresh parsley if desired.

Nutrition Information (Per Serving)

- Calories: 150
- Protein: 3g
- Carbohydrates: 18g
- Dietary Fiber: 4g
- Sugars: 6g
- Fat: 8g
- Saturated Fat: 5g
- Cholesterol: 0mg
- Sodium: 200mg

Servings

- **6 servings**

Cooking Time

- **25 minutes**

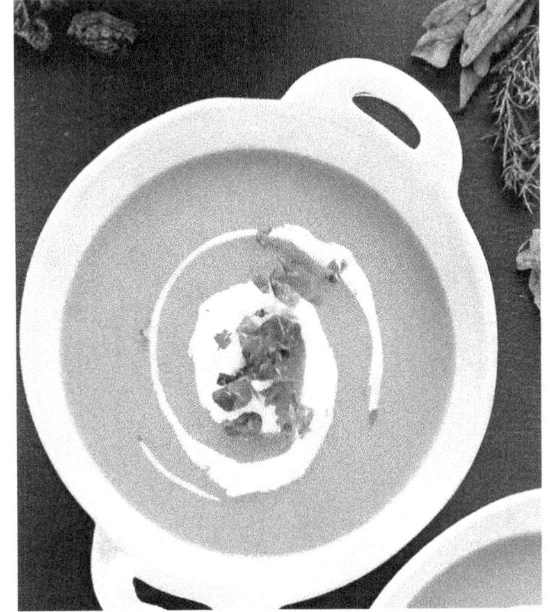

8. Baked Oatmeal

Ingredients

- 2 cups rolled oats
- 1 teaspoon baking powder
- 1 teaspoon ground cinnamon
- 1/4 teaspoon ground nutmeg
- 2 cups almond milk (or any milk of your choice)
- 1/4 cup honey
- 1 large egg
- 1 teaspoon vanilla extract
- 1 cup mixed berries (blueberries, strawberries, raspberries)
- 1/2 cup chopped nuts (optional)

Instructions

1. Preheat the oven to 375°F (190°C) and lightly grease an 8x8-inch baking dish.
2. In a large bowl, combine the rolled oats, baking powder, ground cinnamon, and ground nutmeg.
3. In another bowl, whisk together the almond milk, honey, egg, and vanilla extract.
4. Pour the wet ingredients into the dry ingredients and stir until well combined.
5. Fold in the mixed berries and nuts (if using).
6. Pour the mixture into the prepared baking dish and spread it out evenly.
7. Bake for 35-40 minutes, until the top is golden and the oatmeal is set.
8. Let it cool slightly before serving.

Nutrition Information (Per Serving)

- Calories: 220
- Protein: 6g
- Carbohydrates: 35g
- Dietary Fiber: 5g
- Sugars: 15g
- Fat: 7g
- Saturated Fat: 1g
- Cholesterol: 25mg
- Sodium: 110mg

Servings

- **6 servings**

Cooking Time

- **45 minutes**

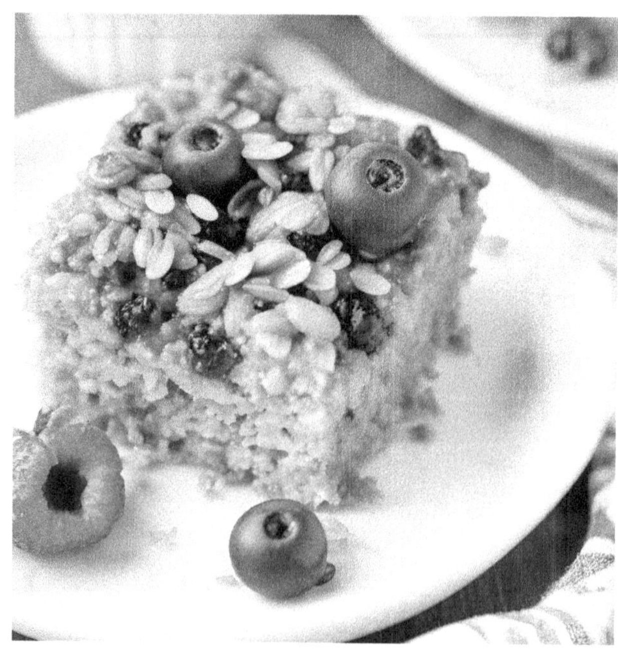

9. Yogurt with Blueberries

Ingredients

- 2 cups plain Greek yogurt
- 1 cup fresh blueberries
- 2 tablespoons honey
- 1/2 teaspoon ground cinnamon
- 1/4 cup granola (optional)

Instructions

1. Divide the Greek yogurt evenly between two bowls.
2. Top each bowl with fresh blueberries.
3. Drizzle with honey and sprinkle with ground cinnamon.
4. Add granola on top if desired.
5. Serve immediately.

Nutrition Information (Per Serving)

- Calories: 180
- Protein: 12g
- Carbohydrates: 25g
- Dietary Fiber: 2g
- Sugars: 18g
- Fat: 4g
- Saturated Fat: 2g
- Cholesterol: 10mg
- Sodium: 70mg

Servings

- **2 servings**

Cooking Time

- **5 minutes**

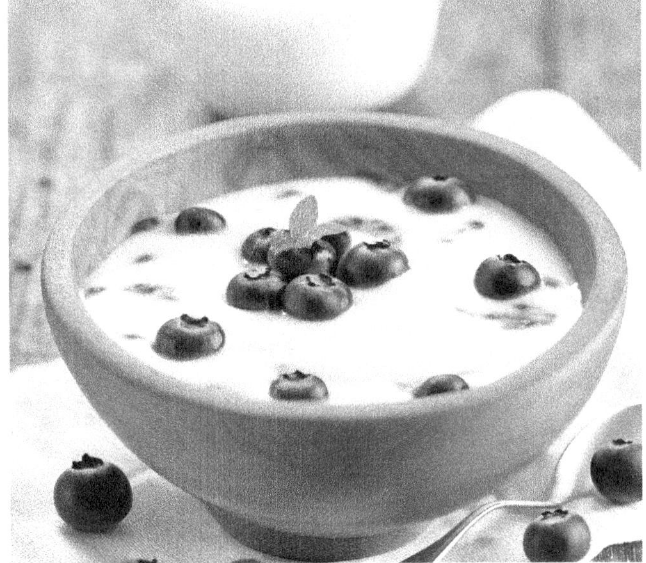

10. Herbal Tea and Rice Cakes

Ingredients

- 2 cups water
- 2 herbal tea bags (e.g., chamomile, ginger, or peppermint)
- 4 rice cakes
- 1/2 cup almond butter or any nut butter
- 1 tablespoon honey
- 1/2 teaspoon ground cinnamon

Instructions

1. Bring the water to a boil in a kettle or pot.
2. Pour the boiling water over the herbal tea bags in a teapot or two cups. Let steep for 5-7 minutes.
3. While the tea is steeping, spread almond butter evenly on each rice cake.
4. Drizzle the rice cakes with honey and sprinkle with ground cinnamon.
5. Serve the rice cakes alongside the herbal tea.

Nutrition Information (Per Serving)

- Calories: 180
- Protein: 5g
- Carbohydrates: 26g
- Dietary Fiber: 3g
- Sugars: 9g
- Fat: 8g
- Saturated Fat: 1g
- Cholesterol: 0mg
- Sodium: 35mg

Servings

- **2 servings**

Cooking Time

- **10 minutes**

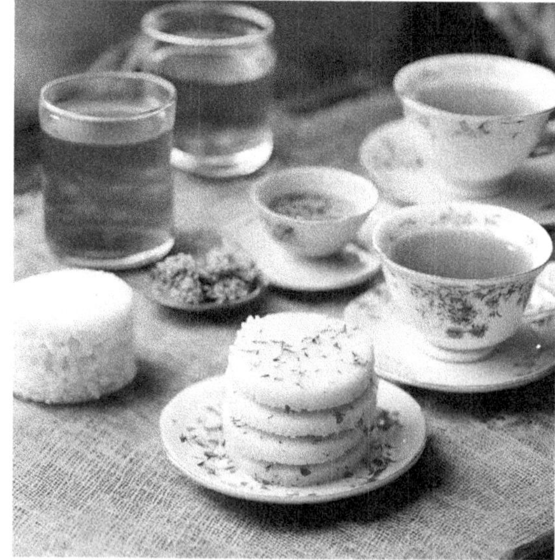

11. Mashed Avocado Bowl

Ingredients

- 2 ripe avocados
- 1/4 cup plain Greek yogurt
- 1 tablespoon lemon juice
- 1/4 teaspoon ground cumin
- 1/4 teaspoon ground paprika
- Whole grain toast or rice cakes (optional)

Instructions

1. Cut the avocados in half, remove the pits, and scoop the flesh into a bowl.
2. Add the Greek yogurt, lemon juice, ground cumin, and ground paprika to the bowl.
3. Mash everything together until smooth and well combined.
4. Serve the mashed avocado mixture in bowls. Optionally, spread it on whole grain toast or rice cakes.

Nutrition Information (Per Serving)

- Calories: 220
- Protein: 4g
- Carbohydrates: 14g
- Dietary Fiber: 9g
- Sugars: 2g
- Fat: 18g
- Saturated Fat: 3g
- Cholesterol: 5mg
- Sodium: 20mg

Servings

- 2 servings

Cooking Time

- **10 minutes**

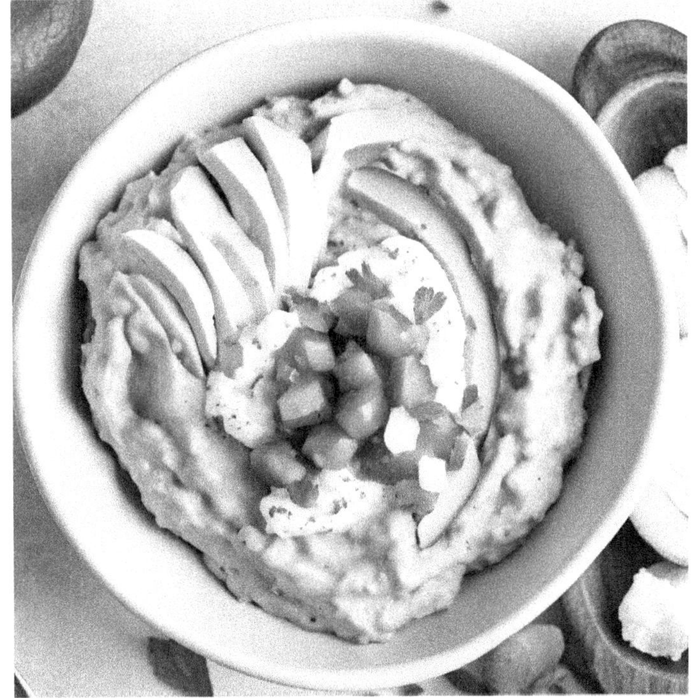

12. Zucchini Bread

Ingredients

- 1 1/2 cups whole wheat flour
- 1 teaspoon baking soda
- 1/2 teaspoon baking powder
- 1 teaspoon ground cinnamon
- 1/2 teaspoon ground nutmeg
- 2 large eggs
- 1/2 cup honey
- 1/2 cup plain Greek yogurt
- 1 teaspoon vanilla extract
- 1 1/2 cups grated zucchini (about 2 medium zucchinis)
- 1/2 cup chopped walnuts (optional)

Instructions

1. Preheat the oven to 350°F (175°C) and grease a 9x5-inch loaf pan.
2. In a large bowl, whisk together the flour, baking soda, baking powder, ground cinnamon, and ground nutmeg.
3. In another bowl, beat the eggs and then add the honey, Greek yogurt, and vanilla extract. Mix well.
4. Add the wet ingredients to the dry ingredients and stir until just combined.
5. Fold in the grated zucchini and walnuts (if using).
6. Pour the batter into the prepared loaf pan and spread it out evenly.
7. Bake for 50-60 minutes, or until a toothpick inserted into the center comes out clean.
8. Let the bread cool in the pan for 10 minutes, then transfer to a wire rack to cool completely.

Nutrition Information (Per Serving)

- Calories: 180
- Protein: 5g
- Carbohydrates: 30g
- Dietary Fiber: 3g
- Sugars: 15g
- Fat: 6g
- Saturated Fat: 1g
- Cholesterol: 35mg
- Sodium: 200mg

Servings

- **10 servings**

Cooking Time

- **70 minutes**

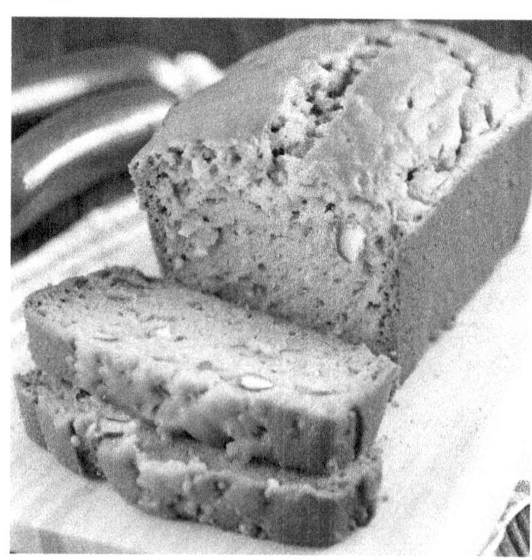

13. Almond Milk Porridge

Ingredients

- 1 cup rolled oats
- 2 cups almond milk (or any milk of your choice)
- 1 tablespoon honey
- 1/2 teaspoon ground cinnamon
- 1/4 teaspoon ground nutmeg
- 1/2 cup sliced almonds
- 1/2 cup fresh or dried berries (optional)

Instructions

1. In a medium saucepan, bring the almond milk to a gentle boil.
2. Stir in the rolled oats and reduce the heat to a simmer. Cook for about 5-7 minutes, stirring occasionally, until the oats are tender and have absorbed most of the liquid.
3. Stir in the honey, ground cinnamon, and ground nutmeg.
4. Serve the porridge in bowls, topped with sliced almonds and berries (if using).

Nutrition Information (Per Serving)

- Calories: 220
- Protein: 6g
- Carbohydrates: 33g
- Dietary Fiber: 5g
- Sugars: 12g
- Fat: 8g
- Saturated Fat: 0.5g
- Cholesterol: 0mg
- Sodium: 60mg

Servings

- 2 servings

Cooking Time

- 10 minutes

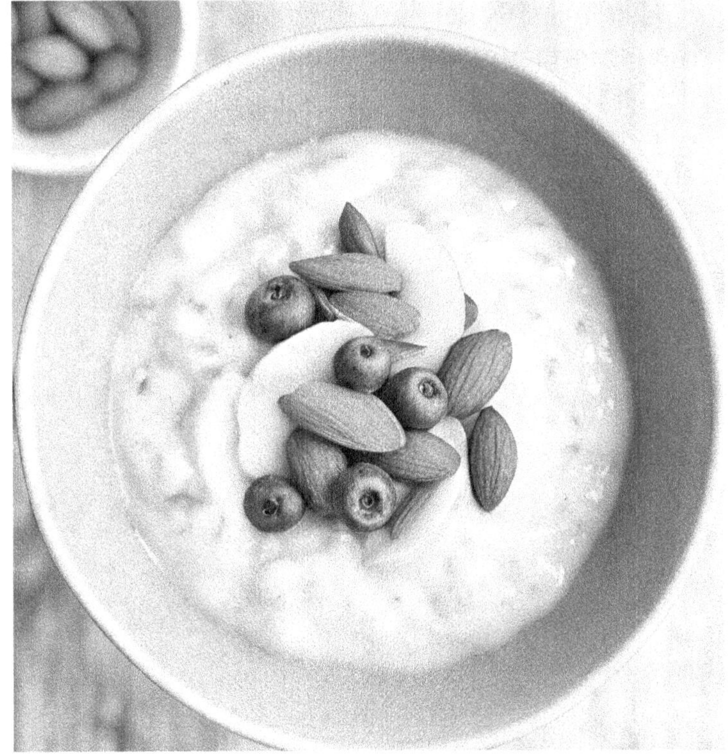

14. Sweet Potato Casserole

Ingredients

- 4 medium sweet potatoes, peeled and cubed
- 1/4 cup almond milk (or any milk of your choice)
- 2 tablespoons honey
- 1 teaspoon vanilla extract
- 1/2 teaspoon ground cinnamon
- 1/4 teaspoon ground nutmeg
- 1/4 cup chopped pecans (optional)

Instructions

1. Preheat the oven to 375°F (190°C) and grease a 9x13-inch baking dish.
2. Boil the sweet potatoes in a large pot of water until tender, about 15-20 minutes.
3. Drain the sweet potatoes and transfer them to a large mixing bowl.
4. Add the almond milk, honey, vanilla extract, ground cinnamon, and ground nutmeg to the sweet potatoes. Mash until smooth.
5. Spread the mashed sweet potato mixture into the prepared baking dish.
6. Sprinkle with chopped pecans if desired.
7. Bake for 25-30 minutes, until the top is slightly browned and the casserole is heated through.
8. Let it cool slightly before serving.

Nutrition Information (Per Serving)

- Calories: 180
- Protein: 2g
- Carbohydrates: 37g
- Dietary Fiber: 5g
- Sugars: 13g
- Fat: 3g
- Saturated Fat: 0g
- Cholesterol: 0mg
- Sodium: 40mg

Servings

- 6 servings

Cooking Time

- **45 minutes**

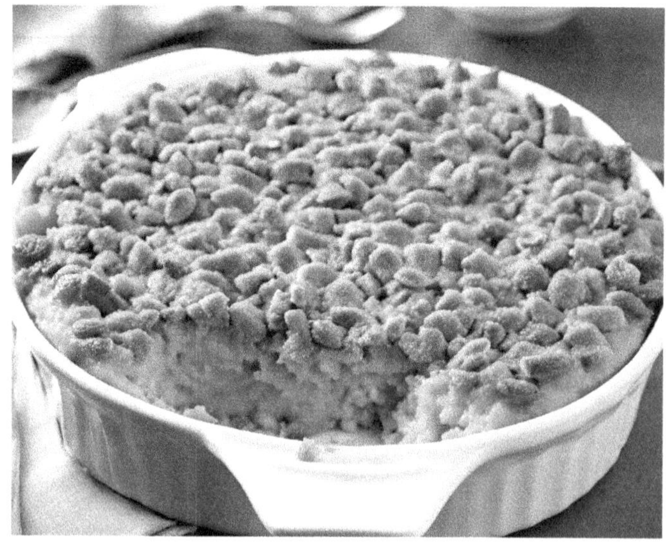

15. Papaya Smoothie

Ingredients

- 1 cup ripe papaya, peeled, seeded, and cubed
- 1 banana
- 1 cup almond milk (or any milk of your choice)
- 1/2 cup Greek yogurt
- 1 tablespoon honey
- 1/2 teaspoon ground cinnamon

Instructions

1. Place the papaya, banana, almond milk, Greek yogurt, honey, and ground cinnamon in a blender.
2. Blend until smooth and creamy.
3. Pour into glasses and serve immediately.

Nutrition Information (Per Serving)

- Calories: 180
- Protein: 5g
- Carbohydrates: 35g
- Dietary Fiber: 4g
- Sugars: 25g
- Fat: 3g
- Saturated Fat: 0.5g
- Cholesterol: 5mg
- Sodium: 50mg

Servings

- **2 servings**

Cooking Time

- **5 minutes**

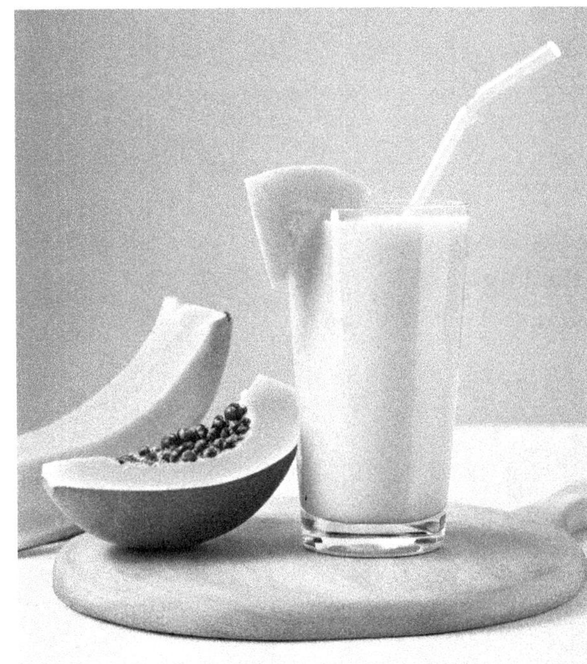

16. Quinoa Breakfast Bowl

Ingredients

- 1 cup quinoa
- 2 cups water
- 1 cup almond milk (or any milk of your choice)
- 1 tablespoon honey
- 1/2 teaspoon ground cinnamon
- 1/4 teaspoon ground nutmeg
- 1/2 cup fresh berries (blueberries, strawberries, raspberries)
- 1/4 cup chopped nuts (optional)

Instructions

1. Rinse the quinoa under cold water until the water runs clear.
2. In a medium saucepan, bring the water to a boil. Add the quinoa, reduce the heat to low, cover, and simmer for about 15 minutes, or until the quinoa is cooked and the water is absorbed.
3. Stir in the almond milk, honey, ground cinnamon, and ground nutmeg. Cook for an additional 5 minutes, stirring occasionally.
4. Serve the quinoa in bowls, topped with fresh berries and chopped nuts (if using).

Nutrition Information (Per Serving)

- Calories: 220
- Protein: 6g
- Carbohydrates: 35g
- Dietary Fiber: 5g
- Sugars: 12g
- Fat: 6g
- Saturated Fat: 0.5g
- Cholesterol: 0mg
- Sodium: 20mg

Servings

- **4 servings**

Cooking Time

- **25 minutes**

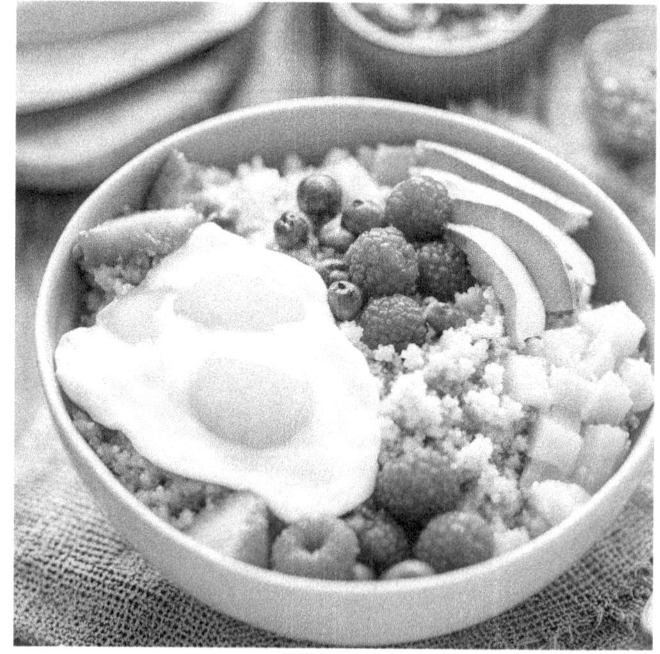

17. Banana Bread

Ingredients

- 2 cups whole wheat flour
- 1 teaspoon baking soda
- 1/2 teaspoon baking powder
- 1 teaspoon ground cinnamon
- 1/4 teaspoon ground nutmeg
- 3 ripe bananas, mashed
- 1/2 cup honey
- 1/4 cup plain Greek yogurt
- 2 large eggs
- 1 teaspoon vanilla extract
- 1/2 cup chopped walnuts (optional)

Instructions

1. Preheat the oven to 350°F (175°C) and lightly grease a 9x5-inch loaf pan.
2. In a large bowl, whisk together the whole wheat flour, baking soda, baking powder, ground cinnamon, and ground nutmeg.
3. In another bowl, mix the mashed bananas, honey, Greek yogurt, eggs, and vanilla extract until well combined.
4. Pour the wet ingredients into the dry ingredients and stir until just combined. Do not overmix.
5. Fold in the chopped walnuts (if using).
6. Pour the batter into the prepared loaf pan and spread it out evenly.
7. Bake for 50-60 minutes, or until a toothpick inserted into the center comes out clean.
8. Let the bread cool in the pan for 10 minutes, then transfer to a wire rack to cool completely.

Nutrition Information (Per Serving)

- Calories: 180
- Protein: 5g
- Carbohydrates: 32g
- Dietary Fiber: 4g
- Sugars: 15g
- Fat: 5g
- Saturated Fat: 1g
- Cholesterol: 35mg
- Sodium: 200mg

Servings

- **10 servings**

Cooking Time

- **70 minutes**

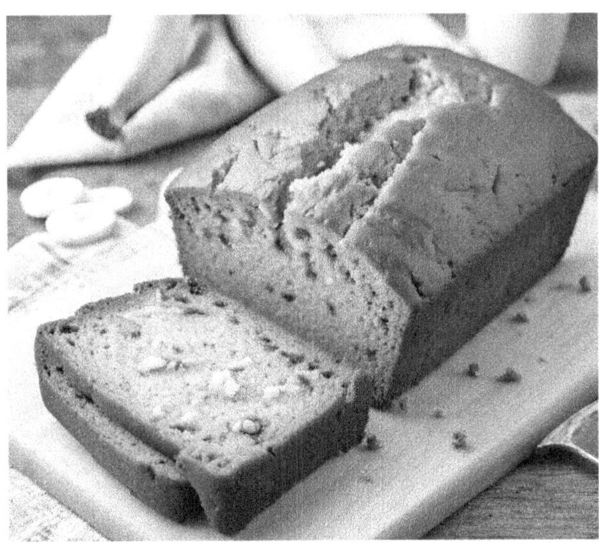

18. Herbal Tea Oatmeal

Ingredients

- 1 cup rolled oats
- 2 cups brewed herbal tea (such as chamomile, ginger, or peppermint)
- 1 tablespoon honey
- 1/2 teaspoon ground cinnamon
- 1/4 teaspoon ground nutmeg
- 1/4 cup chopped nuts (optional)
- 1/2 cup fresh berries (optional)

Instructions

1. Brew the herbal tea and bring it to a gentle boil in a medium saucepan.
2. Stir in the rolled oats, reduce the heat to low, and simmer for about 5-7 minutes, stirring occasionally, until the oats are tender and have absorbed most of the liquid.
3. Stir in the honey, ground cinnamon, and ground nutmeg.
4. Serve the oatmeal in bowls, topped with chopped nuts and fresh berries if desired.

Nutrition Information (Per Serving)

- Calories: 190
- Protein: 5g
- Carbohydrates: 33g
- Dietary Fiber: 4g
- Sugars: 12g
- Fat: 4g
- Saturated Fat: 0.5g
- Cholesterol: 0mg
- Sodium: 20mg

Servings

- **2 servings**

Cooking Time

- **10 minutes**

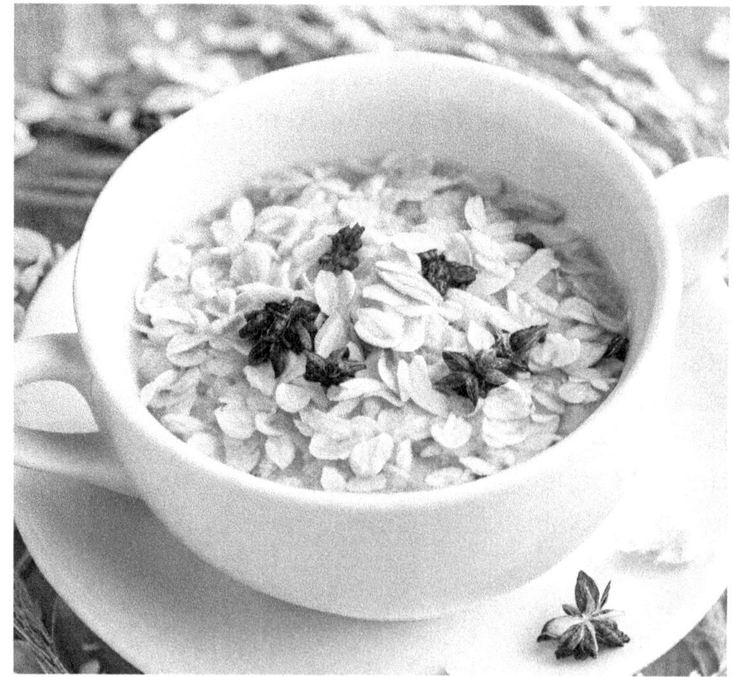

19. Egg White Omelette

Ingredients

- 4 large egg whites
- 1/4 cup almond milk (or any milk of your choice)
- 1/4 teaspoon ground black pepper
- 1/4 teaspoon ground cumin
- 1/2 cup chopped spinach
- 1/4 cup grated low-fat cheese (optional)
- 1 tablespoon olive oil

Instructions

1. In a bowl, whisk together the egg whites, almond milk, ground black pepper, and ground cumin until well combined.
2. Heat the olive oil in a non-stick skillet over medium heat.
3. Pour the egg white mixture into the skillet and cook for about 2-3 minutes, until the edges start to set.
4. Sprinkle the chopped spinach and grated cheese (if using) over one half of the omelette.
5. Fold the other half of the omelette over the filling and cook for another 2-3 minutes, until the eggs are fully set and the cheese is melted.
6. Slide the omelette onto a plate and serve immediately.

Nutrition Information (Per Serving)

- Calories: 120
- Protein: 15g
- Carbohydrates: 2g
- Dietary Fiber: 1g
- Sugars: 1g
- Fat: 5g
- Saturated Fat: 1g
- Cholesterol: 0mg
- Sodium: 150mg

Servings

- 2 servings

Cooking Time

- 10 minutes

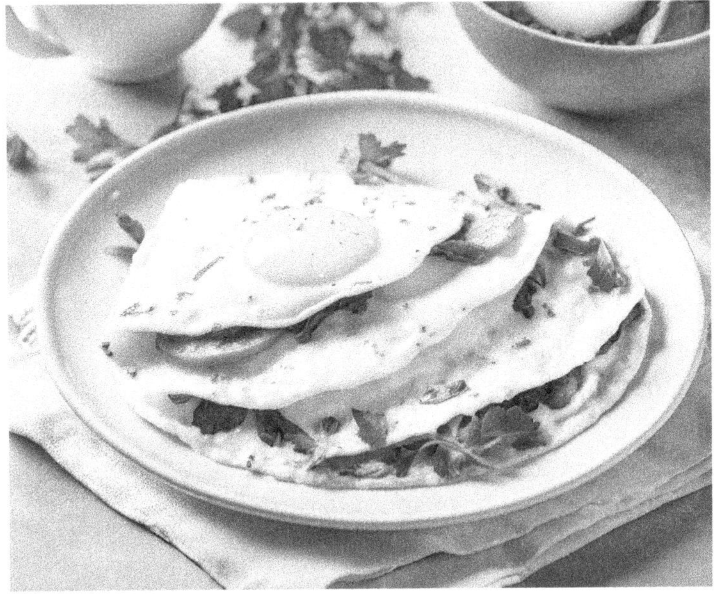

20. Buckwheat Pancakes

Ingredients

- 1 cup buckwheat flour
- 1 tablespoon baking powder
- 1/2 teaspoon ground cinnamon
- 1/4 teaspoon ground nutmeg
- 1 cup almond milk (or any milk of your choice)
- 1 large egg
- 1 tablespoon honey
- 1 teaspoon vanilla extract
- 2 tablespoons olive oil (for cooking)

Instructions

1. In a large bowl, mix the buckwheat flour, baking powder, ground cinnamon, and ground nutmeg.
2. In another bowl, whisk together the almond milk, egg, honey, and vanilla extract.
3. Pour the wet ingredients into the dry ingredients and stir until just combined. Do not overmix.
4. Heat a non-stick skillet or griddle over medium heat and lightly coat with olive oil.
5. Pour 1/4 cup of batter onto the skillet for each pancake.
6. Cook until bubbles form on the surface and the edges look set, about 2-3 minutes. Flip and cook for another 2-3 minutes until golden brown.
7. Serve warm with additional honey or fresh fruit if desired.

Nutrition Information (Per Serving)

- Calories: 150
- Protein: 4g
- Carbohydrates: 22g
- Dietary Fiber: 3g
- Sugars: 6g
- Fat: 6g
- Saturated Fat: 1g
- Cholesterol: 35mg
- Sodium: 190mg

Servings

- **4 servings**

Cooking Time

- **20 minutes**

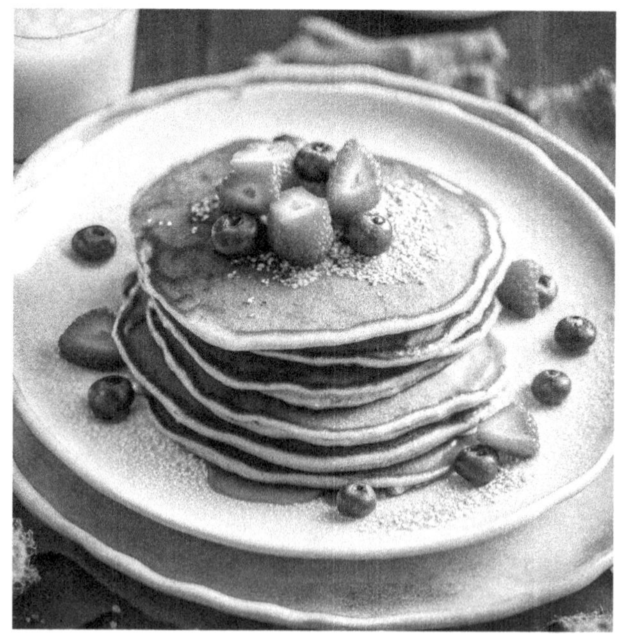

21. Chia Seed Pudding

Ingredients

- 1/4 cup chia seeds
- 1 cup almond milk (or any milk of your choice)
- 1 tablespoon honey
- 1/2 teaspoon vanilla extract
- 1/4 teaspoon ground cinnamon
- Fresh berries or sliced fruit for topping (optional)

Instructions

1. In a bowl or jar, combine the chia seeds, almond milk, honey, vanilla extract, and ground cinnamon. Stir well to combine.
2. Let the mixture sit for about 5 minutes, then stir again to prevent the chia seeds from clumping.
3. Cover the bowl or jar and refrigerate for at least 2 hours, or overnight, until the pudding has thickened.
4. Stir the pudding before serving and top with fresh berries or sliced fruit if desired.

Nutrition Information (Per Serving)

- Calories: 180
- Protein: 5g
- Carbohydrates: 20g
- Dietary Fiber: 10g
- Sugars: 9g
- Fat: 9g
- Saturated Fat: 0.5g
- Cholesterol: 0mg
- Sodium: 50mg

Servings

- 2 servings

Cooking Time

- 5 minutes prep, 2 hours refrigeration

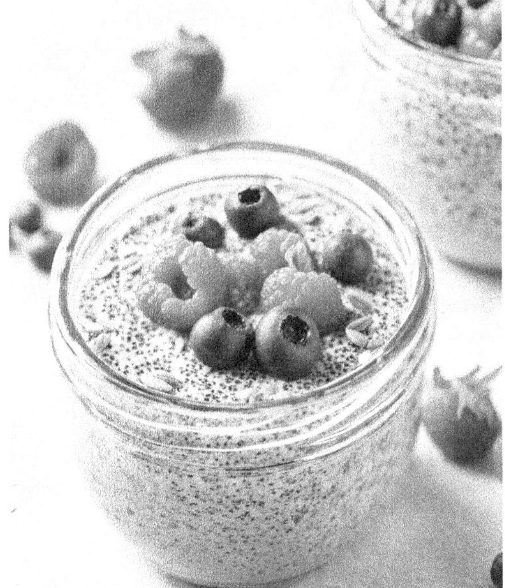

22. Apple Cinnamon Porridge

Ingredients

- 1 cup rolled oats
- 2 cups almond milk (or any milk of your choice)
- 1 apple, peeled, cored, and diced
- 1 tablespoon honey
- 1 teaspoon ground cinnamon
- 1/4 teaspoon ground nutmeg
- 1/4 cup chopped nuts (optional)

Instructions

1. In a medium saucepan, bring the almond milk to a gentle boil.
2. Stir in the rolled oats, diced apple, ground cinnamon, and ground nutmeg. Reduce the heat to a simmer and cook for about 5-7 minutes, stirring occasionally, until the oats are tender and have absorbed most of the liquid.
3. Stir in the honey.
4. Serve the porridge in bowls, topped with chopped nuts if desired.

Nutrition Information (Per Serving)

- Calories: 220
- Protein: 5g
- Carbohydrates: 40g
- Dietary Fiber: 6g
- Sugars: 15g
- Fat: 6g
- Saturated Fat: 0.5g
- Cholesterol: 0mg
- Sodium: 60mg

Servings

- **2 servings**

Cooking Time

- **10 minutes**

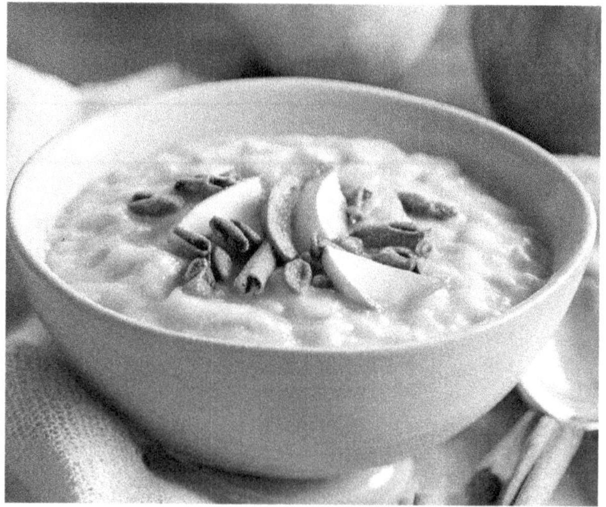

23. Millet Porridge

Ingredients

- 1 cup millet
- 3 cups water
- 1 cup almond milk (or any milk of your choice)
- 1 tablespoon honey
- 1 teaspoon ground cinnamon
- 1/4 teaspoon ground nutmeg
- 1/4 cup chopped nuts (optional)
- Fresh berries for topping (optional)

Instructions

1. Rinse the millet under cold water.
2. In a medium saucepan, bring the water to a boil. Add the millet, reduce the heat to low, cover, and simmer for about 20 minutes, or until the millet is tender and the water is absorbed.
3. Stir in the almond milk, honey, ground cinnamon, and ground nutmeg. Cook for an additional 5 minutes, stirring occasionally.
4. Serve the porridge in bowls, topped with chopped nuts and fresh berries if desired.

Nutrition Information (Per Serving)

- Calories: 210
- Protein: 5g
- Carbohydrates: 35g
- Dietary Fiber: 5g
- Sugars: 10g
- Fat: 6g
- Saturated Fat: 0.5g
- Cholesterol: 0mg
- Sodium: 10mg

Servings

- **4 servings**

Cooking Time

- **30 minutes**

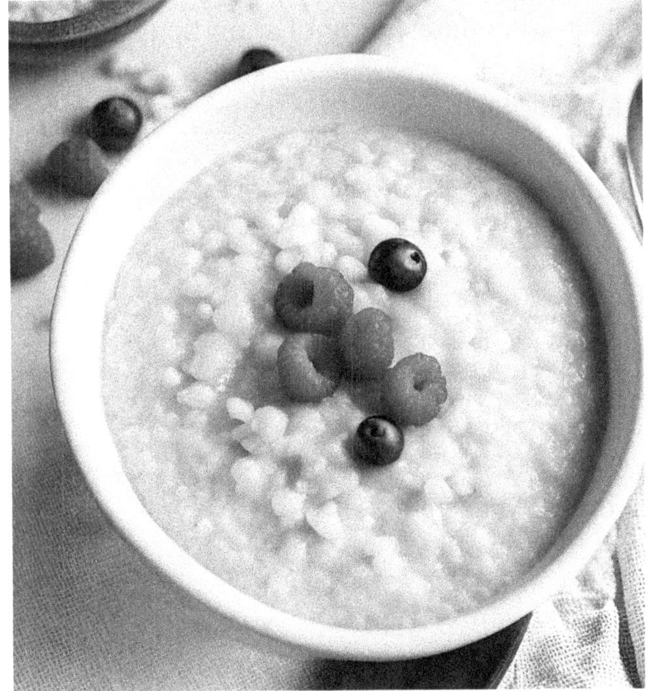

24. Banana Muffins

Ingredients

- 1 1/2 cups whole wheat flour
- 1 teaspoon baking soda
- 1 teaspoon ground cinnamon
- 1/4 teaspoon ground nutmeg
- 3 ripe bananas, mashed
- 1/3 cup honey
- 1/4 cup plain Greek yogurt
- 1 large egg
- 1 teaspoon vanilla extract
- 1/4 cup chopped walnuts (optional)

Instructions

1. Preheat the oven to 350°F (175°C) and line a muffin tin with paper liners.
2. In a large bowl, whisk together the whole wheat flour, baking soda, ground cinnamon, and ground nutmeg.
3. In another bowl, mix the mashed bananas, honey, Greek yogurt, egg, and vanilla extract until well combined.
4. Pour the wet ingredients into the dry ingredients and stir until just combined. Do not overmix.
5. Fold in the chopped walnuts (if using).
6. Divide the batter evenly among the muffin cups.
7. Bake for 18-20 minutes, or until a toothpick inserted into the center of a muffin comes out clean.
8. Allow the muffins to cool in the tin for 5 minutes, then transfer to a wire rack to cool completely.

Nutrition Information (Per Serving)

- Calories: 150
- Protein: 4g
- Carbohydrates: 30g
- Dietary Fiber: 4g
- Sugars: 12g
- Fat: 4g
- Saturated Fat: 0.5g
- Cholesterol: 20mg
- Sodium: 150mg

Servings

- **12 muffins**

Cooking Time

- **25 minutes**

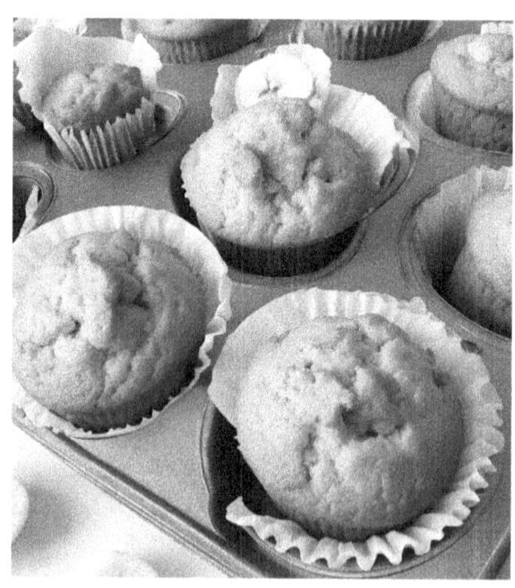

25. Sweet Rice Balls

Ingredients

- 1 cup glutinous rice
- 2 cups water
- 1/4 cup honey
- 1/2 cup shredded coconut
- 1/2 teaspoon ground cinnamon
- 1/4 teaspoon ground nutmeg
- Fresh berries for serving (optional)

Instructions

1. Rinse the glutinous rice under cold water until the water runs clear.
2. In a medium saucepan, combine the rice and water. Bring to a boil, then reduce the heat to low, cover, and simmer for 15-20 minutes, or until the rice is tender and the water is absorbed.
3. Remove the rice from the heat and let it cool slightly.
4. Stir in the honey, shredded coconut, ground cinnamon, and ground nutmeg.
5. Wet your hands with water to prevent sticking and shape the rice mixture into small balls.
6. Serve the sweet rice balls with fresh berries if desired.

Nutrition Information (Per Serving)

- Calories: 150
- Protein: 2g
- Carbohydrates: 32g
- Dietary Fiber: 2g
- Sugars: 12g
- Fat: 2g
- Saturated Fat: 1g
- Cholesterol: 0mg
- Sodium: 10mg

Servings

- **8 servings**

Cooking Time

- **30 minutes**

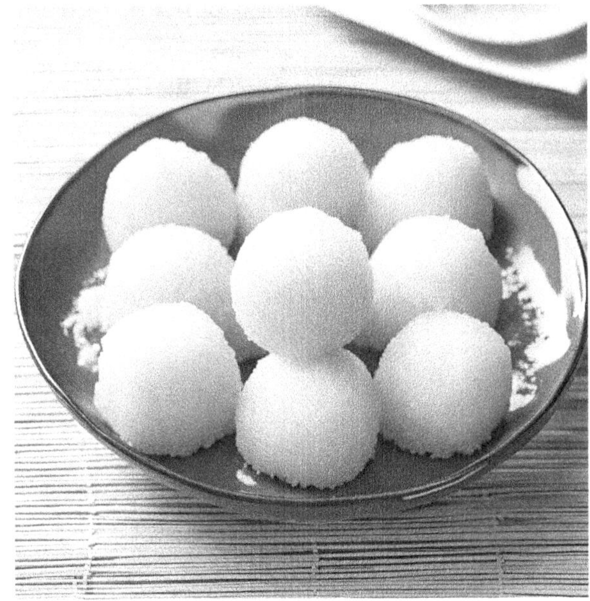

Fish & Seafood Recipes

1. Tilapia Piccata
Ingredients
- 4 tilapia fillets
- 1/4 cup whole wheat flour
- 1 tablespoon olive oil
- 1/4 cup low-sodium chicken broth
- 2 tablespoons lemon juice
- 2 tablespoons capers, drained
- 1/4 cup fresh parsley, chopped

Instructions
1. Lightly coat the tilapia fillets with whole wheat flour, shaking off any excess.
2. In a large skillet, heat the olive oil over medium heat.
3. Add the tilapia fillets to the skillet and cook for 3-4 minutes on each side, until the fish is golden brown and cooked through. Remove the fish from the skillet and keep warm.
4. In the same skillet, add the chicken broth, lemon juice, and capers. Cook for 2-3 minutes, stirring occasionally, until the sauce thickens slightly.
5. Return the tilapia fillets to the skillet and spoon the sauce over the top. Cook for an additional 1-2 minutes.
6. Sprinkle with fresh parsley before serving.

Nutrition Information (Per Serving)
- Calories: 200
- Protein: 26g
- Carbohydrates: 7g
- Dietary Fiber: 1g
- Sugars: 0g
- Fat: 7g
- Saturated Fat: 1g
- Cholesterol: 55mg
- Sodium: 220mg

Servings
- **4 servings**

Cooking Time
- **20 minutes**

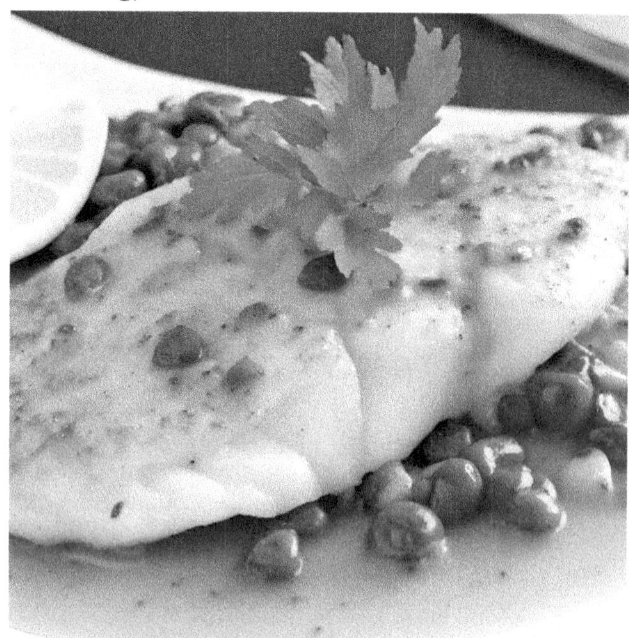

2. Shrimp Coconut Curry

Ingredients

- 1 pound large shrimp, peeled and deveined
- 1 tablespoon olive oil
- 1 cup coconut milk
- 1/2 cup low-sodium vegetable broth
- 1 tablespoon curry powder
- 1 teaspoon ground turmeric
- 1 teaspoon ground ginger
- 2 cups spinach, chopped
- 1/4 cup fresh cilantro, chopped

Instructions

1. In a large skillet, heat the olive oil over medium heat.
2. Add the shrimp to the skillet and cook for 2-3 minutes on each side, until pink and opaque. Remove the shrimp from the skillet and set aside.
3. In the same skillet, add the coconut milk, vegetable broth, curry powder, ground turmeric, and ground ginger. Stir to combine and bring to a simmer.
4. Add the chopped spinach to the skillet and cook for 2-3 minutes, until wilted.
5. Return the shrimp to the skillet and cook for an additional 2-3 minutes, until heated through.
6. Garnish with fresh cilantro before serving.

Nutrition Information (Per Serving)

- Calories: 300
- Protein: 24g
- Carbohydrates: 8g
- Dietary Fiber: 2g
- Sugars: 2g
- Fat: 20g
- Saturated Fat: 15g
- Cholesterol: 190mg
- Sodium: 320mg

Servings

- **4 servings**

Cooking Time

- **25 minutes**

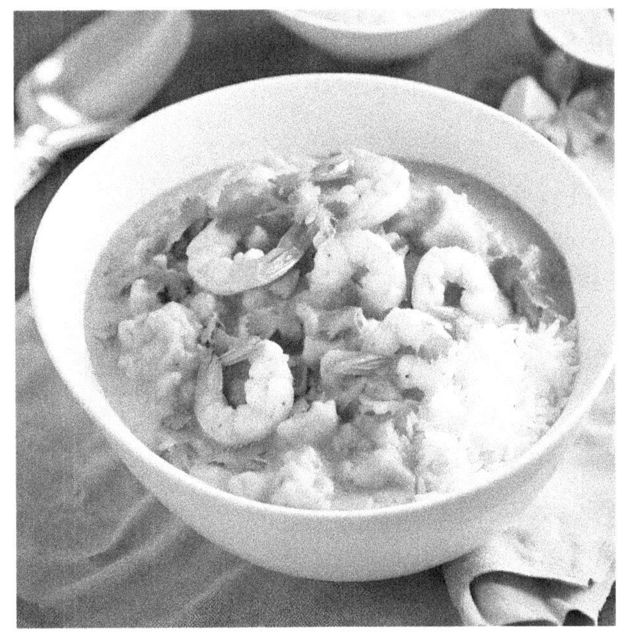

3. Fried Sole with Oatmeal

Ingredients

- 4 sole fillets
- 1/2 cup rolled oats
- 1/4 cup whole wheat flour
- 1 large egg, beaten
- 2 tablespoons olive oil
- 1/4 cup fresh parsley, chopped
- Lemon wedges for serving

Instructions

1. In a food processor, pulse the rolled oats until they resemble coarse breadcrumbs.
2. Set up a breading station with three shallow dishes: one with the whole wheat flour, one with the beaten egg, and one with the ground oats.
3. Dredge each sole fillet in the flour, then dip in the egg, and finally coat with the ground oats.
4. In a large skillet, heat the olive oil over medium heat.
5. Add the sole fillets to the skillet and cook for 3-4 minutes on each side, until golden brown and cooked through.
6. Sprinkle with fresh parsley before serving. Serve with lemon wedges.

Nutrition Information (Per Serving)

- Calories: 250
- Protein: 25g
- Carbohydrates: 15g
- Dietary Fiber: 2g
- Sugars: 0g
- Fat: 10g
- Saturated Fat: 1.5g
- Cholesterol: 85mg
- Sodium: 150mg

Servings

- **4 servings**

Cooking Time

- **20 minutes**

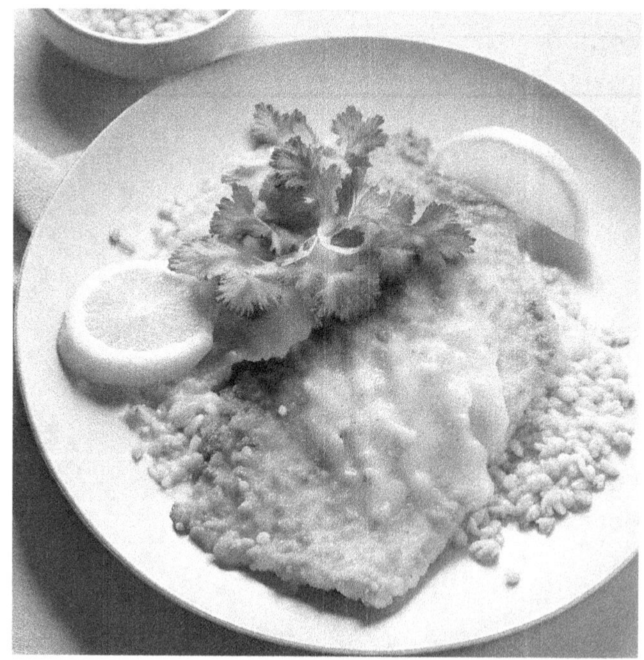

4. Creamy Shrimp Risotto

Ingredients

- 1 cup Arborio rice
- 1 tablespoon olive oil
- 1 pound large shrimp, peeled and deveined
- 1/2 cup low-sodium vegetable broth
- 1/2 cup coconut milk
- 4 cups low-sodium chicken broth, kept warm
- 1/2 teaspoon ground turmeric
- 1/4 cup Parmesan cheese, grated (optional)
- 1/4 cup fresh parsley, chopped

Instructions

1. In a large skillet, heat the olive oil over medium heat. Add the Arborio rice and cook for 2-3 minutes, stirring constantly, until the rice is lightly toasted.
2. Add 1/2 cup of the warm chicken broth to the skillet, stirring constantly until the liquid is absorbed.
3. Continue adding the warm chicken broth 1/2 cup at a time, stirring constantly and allowing the liquid to be absorbed before adding more, until the rice is creamy and cooked through (about 20-25 minutes).
4. In a separate skillet, cook the shrimp over medium heat for 2-3 minutes on each side, until pink and opaque. Remove from heat and set aside.
5. Once the risotto is creamy, stir in the vegetable broth, coconut milk, and ground turmeric. Cook for an additional 2-3 minutes.
6. Add the cooked shrimp and Parmesan cheese (if using) to the risotto, stirring gently to combine.
7. Garnish with fresh parsley before serving.

Nutrition Information (Per Serving)

- Calories: 350
- Protein: 25g
- Carbohydrates: 45g
- Dietary Fiber: 2g
- Sugars: 3g
- Fat: 10g
- Saturated Fat: 6g
- Cholesterol: 190mg
- Sodium: 350mg

Servings

- **4 servings**

Cooking Time

- **30 minutes**

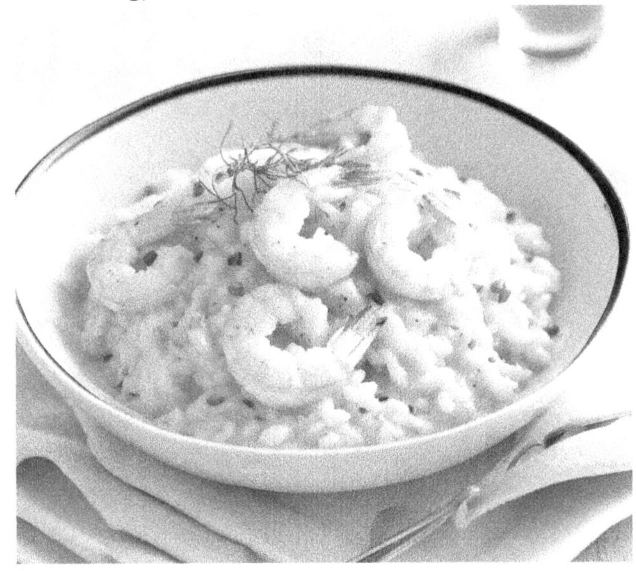

5. Tuna Salad with Avocado

Ingredients

- 2 cans (5 oz each) tuna in water, drained
- 1 large avocado, diced
- 1/4 cup plain Greek yogurt
- 1 tablespoon lemon juice
- 1/4 cup chopped celery
- 1/4 cup chopped fresh parsley
- 1/2 teaspoon ground cumin
- Whole grain crackers or lettuce leaves for serving

Instructions

1. In a large bowl, combine the drained tuna, diced avocado, Greek yogurt, lemon juice, chopped celery, chopped parsley, and ground cumin.
2. Mix gently until well combined.
3. Serve the tuna salad with whole grain crackers or on lettuce leaves.

Nutrition Information (Per Serving)

- Calories: 250
- Protein: 25g
- Carbohydrates: 10g
- Dietary Fiber: 5g
- Sugars: 1g
- Fat: 12g
- Saturated Fat: 2g
- Cholesterol: 40mg
- Sodium: 320mg

Servings

- **4 servings**

Cooking Time

- **10 minutes**

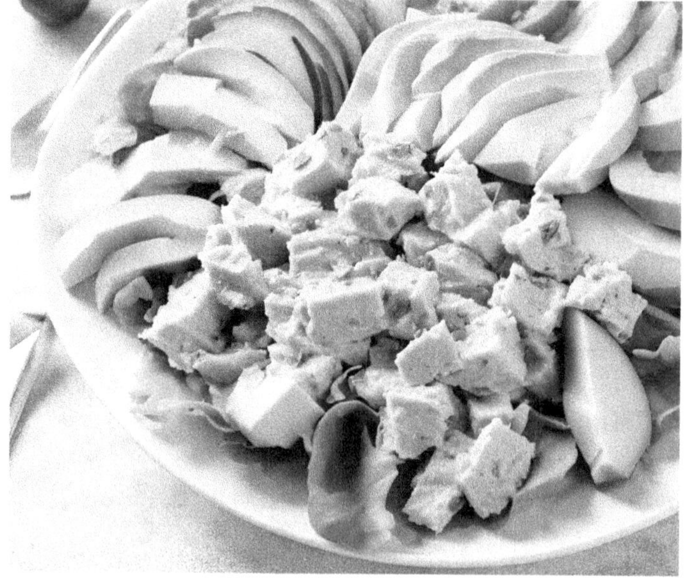

6. Foil-Baked Trout with Vegetables

Ingredients

- 4 trout fillets
- 2 cups sliced zucchini
- 2 cups sliced carrots
- 2 tablespoons olive oil
- 1 tablespoon lemon juice
- 1 teaspoon dried thyme
- 1/4 teaspoon ground black pepper
- Fresh parsley for garnish (optional)

Instructions

1. Preheat the oven to 375°F (190°C).
2. Cut four large pieces of aluminum foil. Place a trout fillet in the center of each piece of foil.
3. Divide the sliced zucchini and carrots evenly among the foil packets, placing the vegetables around the trout fillets.
4. Drizzle each packet with olive oil and lemon juice. Sprinkle with dried thyme and ground black pepper.
5. Fold the foil over the trout and vegetables to create a sealed packet.
6. Place the foil packets on a baking sheet and bake for 20-25 minutes, until the trout is cooked through and the vegetables are tender.
7. Carefully open the foil packets and garnish with fresh parsley if desired before serving.

Nutrition Information (Per Serving)

- Calories: 280
- Protein: 25g
- Carbohydrates: 10g
- Dietary Fiber: 3g
- Sugars: 5g
- Fat: 15g
- Saturated Fat: 2g
- Cholesterol: 55mg
- Sodium: 120mg

Servings

- **4 servings**

Cooking Time

- **30 minutes**

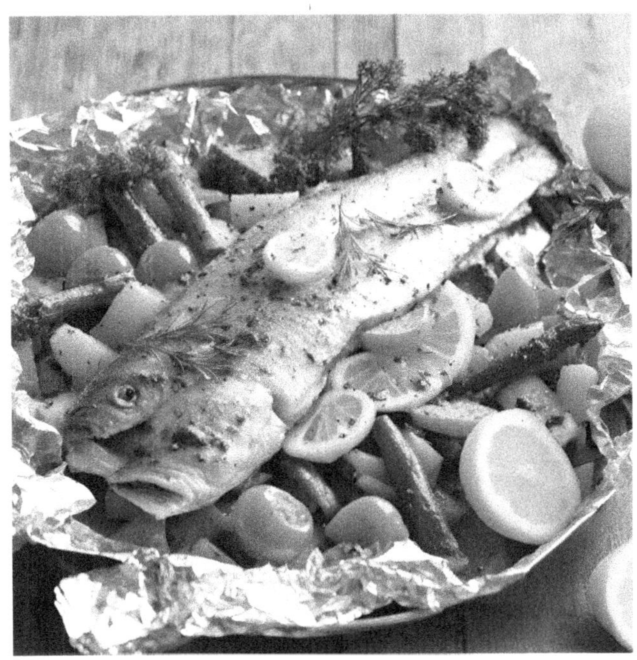

7. Oven-Baked Perch

Ingredients

- 4 perch fillets
- 2 tablespoons olive oil
- 1/4 cup whole wheat bread crumbs
- 1/4 cup grated Parmesan cheese
- 1 teaspoon dried oregano
- 1/2 teaspoon ground paprika
- Lemon wedges for serving

Instructions

1. Preheat the oven to 400°F (200°C) and line a baking sheet with parchment paper.
2. In a small bowl, mix the whole wheat bread crumbs, grated Parmesan cheese, dried oregano, and ground paprika.
3. Brush each perch fillet with olive oil and then coat with the bread crumb mixture.
4. Place the coated fillets on the prepared baking sheet.
5. Bake for 12-15 minutes, or until the fish is golden brown and cooked through.
6. Serve with lemon wedges.

Nutrition Information (Per Serving)

- Calories: 210
- Protein: 28g
- Carbohydrates: 7g
- Dietary Fiber: 1g
- Sugars: 0g
- Fat: 8g
- Saturated Fat: 2g
- Cholesterol: 70mg
- Sodium: 220mg

Servings

- **4 servings**

Cooking Time

- **20 minutes**

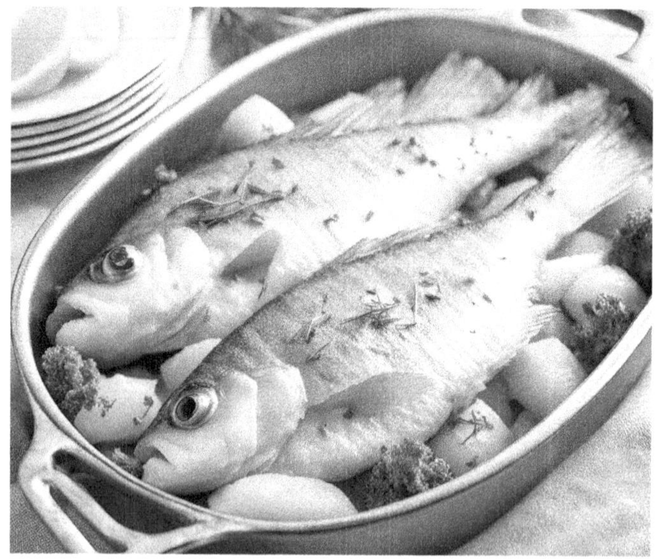

8. Salmon Pasta with Peas

Ingredients

- 8 oz whole wheat pasta
- 1 pound salmon fillet, skin removed and cut into cubes
- 1 cup frozen peas
- 1/2 cup low-sodium vegetable broth
- 1/2 cup plain Greek yogurt
- 1 tablespoon olive oil
- 1 tablespoon lemon juice
- 1 teaspoon dried dill
- 1/4 teaspoon ground black pepper

Instructions

1. Cook the whole wheat pasta according to package instructions. Drain and set aside.
2. In a large skillet, heat the olive oil over medium heat. Add the salmon cubes and cook for 4-5 minutes, until the salmon is cooked through.
3. Add the vegetable broth, frozen peas, Greek yogurt, lemon juice, dried dill, and ground black pepper to the skillet. Stir to combine and cook for 2-3 minutes until the peas are heated through.
4. Add the cooked pasta to the skillet and toss to coat evenly with the sauce.
5. Serve immediately.

Nutrition Information (Per Serving)

- Calories: 350
- Protein: 30g
- Carbohydrates: 40g
- Dietary Fiber: 6g
- Sugars: 3g
- Fat: 10g
- Saturated Fat: 2g
- Cholesterol: 55mg
- Sodium: 150mg

Servings

- **4 servings**

Cooking Time

- **20 minutes**

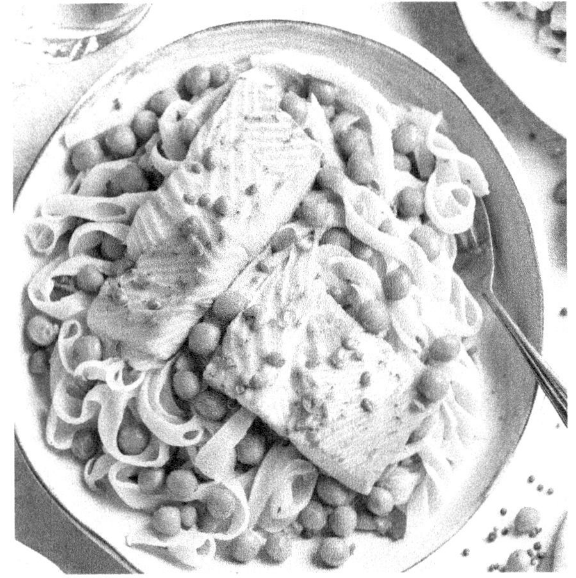

9. Seafood Paella

Ingredients

- 1 cup Arborio rice
- 1 tablespoon olive oil
- 1/2 pound shrimp, peeled and deveined
- 1/2 pound mussels, scrubbed and debearded
- 1/2 pound squid, cleaned and sliced into rings
- 1 cup low-sodium chicken broth
- 1 cup low-sodium vegetable broth
- 1/2 teaspoon ground turmeric
- 1/2 teaspoon ground paprika
- 1 cup frozen peas
- 1/4 cup fresh parsley, chopped

Instructions

1. In a large skillet or paella pan, heat the olive oil over medium heat.
2. Add the Arborio rice and cook for 2-3 minutes, stirring constantly, until the rice is lightly toasted.
3. Add the chicken broth, vegetable broth, ground turmeric, and ground paprika. Stir to combine and bring to a simmer.
4. Arrange the shrimp, mussels, and squid over the rice. Cover and cook for 15-20 minutes, or until the rice is tender and the seafood is cooked through.
5. Stir in the frozen peas and cook for an additional 2-3 minutes.
6. Garnish with fresh parsley before serving.

Nutrition Information (Per Serving)

- Calories: 320
- Protein: 25g
- Carbohydrates: 40g
- Dietary Fiber: 3g
- Sugars: 2g
- Fat: 8g
- Saturated Fat: 1g
- Cholesterol: 150mg
- Sodium: 400mg

Servings

- **4 servings**

Cooking Time

- **30 minutes**

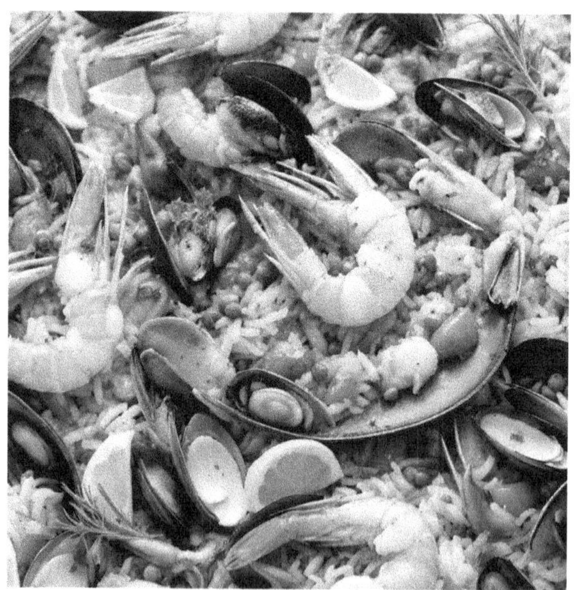

10. Broiled Scallops

Ingredients

- 1 pound sea scallops
- 2 tablespoons olive oil
- 1 tablespoon lemon juice
- 1/2 teaspoon ground paprika
- 1/4 teaspoon ground black pepper
- Fresh parsley for garnish (optional)

Instructions

1. Preheat the broiler and line a baking sheet with aluminum foil.
2. Pat the scallops dry with paper towels and place them on the prepared baking sheet.
3. In a small bowl, whisk together the olive oil, lemon juice, ground paprika, and ground black pepper.
4. Brush the mixture over the scallops.
5. Broil the scallops for 6-8 minutes, turning once halfway through, until they are golden and opaque.
6. Garnish with fresh parsley before serving.

Nutrition Information (Per Serving)

- Calories: 210
- Protein: 24g
- Carbohydrates: 3g
- Dietary Fiber: 0g
- Sugars: 0g
- Fat: 12g
- Saturated Fat: 2g
- Cholesterol: 40mg
- Sodium: 370mg

Servings

- **4 servings**

Cooking Time

- **15 minutes**

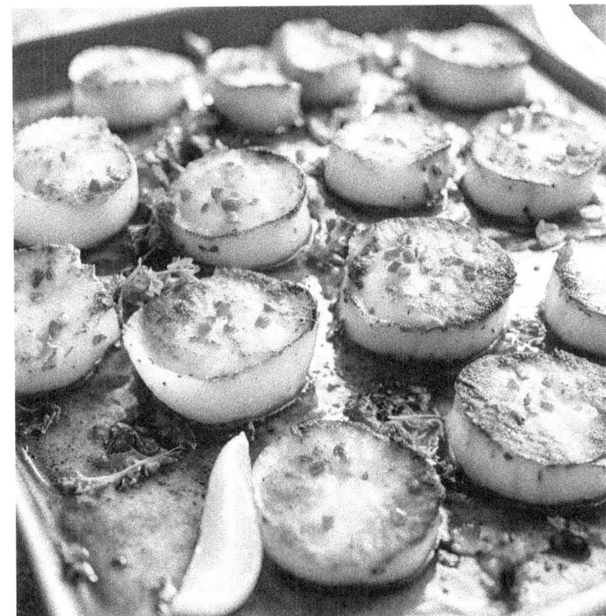

11. Haddock in Parchment

Ingredients

- 4 haddock fillets
- 2 cups thinly sliced zucchini
- 2 cups thinly sliced carrots
- 2 tablespoons olive oil
- 1 tablespoon lemon juice
- 1 teaspoon dried thyme
- 1/4 teaspoon ground black pepper

Instructions

1. Preheat the oven to 375°F (190°C).
2. Cut four large pieces of parchment paper. Place a haddock fillet in the center of each piece of parchment.
3. Divide the sliced zucchini and carrots evenly among the parchment packets, placing the vegetables around the haddock fillets.
4. Drizzle each packet with olive oil and lemon juice. Sprinkle with dried thyme and ground black pepper.
5. Fold the parchment paper over the haddock and vegetables to create a sealed packet.
6. Place the parchment packets on a baking sheet and bake for 20-25 minutes, until the haddock is cooked through and the vegetables are tender.
7. Serve immediately.

Nutrition Information (Per Serving)

- Calories: 220
- Protein: 27g
- Carbohydrates: 7g
- Dietary Fiber: 2g
- Sugars: 4g
- Fat: 9g
- Saturated Fat: 1.5g
- Cholesterol: 75mg
- Sodium: 140mg

Servings

- **4 servings**

Cooking Time

- **30 minutes**

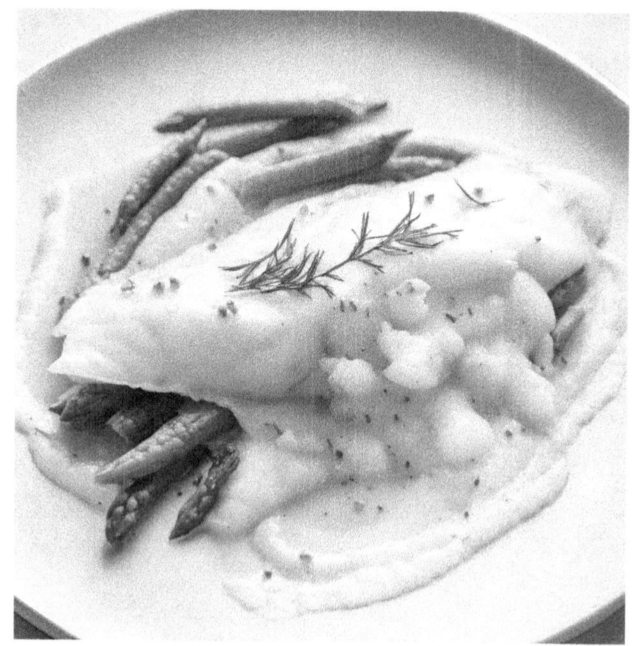

12. Basil Shrimp with Fettuccine

Ingredients

- 8 oz whole wheat fettuccine
- 1 pound large shrimp, peeled and deveined
- 2 tablespoons olive oil
- 1/2 cup low-sodium vegetable broth
- 1/2 cup coconut milk
- 1 teaspoon dried basil
- 1/4 teaspoon ground black pepper
- 1/4 cup fresh basil, chopped

Instructions

1. Cook the fettuccine according to package instructions. Drain and set aside.
2. In a large skillet, heat the olive oil over medium heat. Add the shrimp and cook for 2-3 minutes on each side, until pink and opaque. Remove the shrimp from the skillet and set aside.
3. In the same skillet, add the vegetable broth, coconut milk, dried basil, and ground black pepper. Stir to combine and bring to a simmer.
4. Return the shrimp to the skillet and cook for an additional 2-3 minutes, until heated through.
5. Add the cooked fettuccine to the skillet and toss to coat with the sauce.
6. Serve immediately, garnished with fresh basil.

Nutrition Information (Per Serving)

- Calories: 350
- Protein: 28g
- Carbohydrates: 40g
- Dietary Fiber: 5g
- Sugars: 2g
- Fat: 12g
- Saturated Fat: 6g
- Cholesterol: 190mg
- Sodium: 300mg

Servings

- **4 servings**

Cooking Time

- **20 minutes**

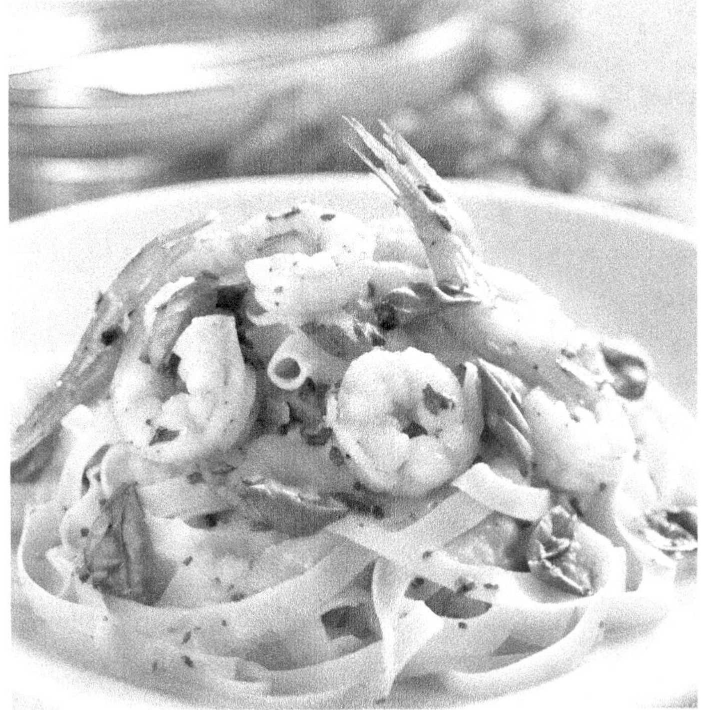

13. Crab Stuffed Mushrooms

Ingredients

- 1 pound large white mushrooms, stems removed
- 1 cup lump crab meat
- 1/4 cup plain Greek yogurt
- 1/4 cup whole wheat bread crumbs
- 1 tablespoon lemon juice
- 1 teaspoon dried dill
- 1/4 teaspoon ground black pepper
- 1/4 cup grated Parmesan cheese (optional)

Instructions

1. Preheat the oven to 375°F (190°C) and line a baking sheet with parchment paper.
2. In a bowl, combine the crab meat, Greek yogurt, whole wheat bread crumbs, lemon juice, dried dill, and ground black pepper. Mix until well combined.
3. Stuff each mushroom cap with the crab mixture and place them on the prepared baking sheet.
4. Sprinkle with grated Parmesan cheese if desired.
5. Bake for 15-20 minutes, until the mushrooms are tender and the filling is golden.
6. Serve immediately.

Nutrition Information (Per Serving)

- Calories: 150
- Protein: 15g
- Carbohydrates: 10g
- Dietary Fiber: 2g
- Sugars: 2g
- Fat: 6g
- Saturated Fat: 2g
- Cholesterol: 60mg
- Sodium: 300mg

Servings

- **4 servings**

Cooking Time

- **25 minutes**

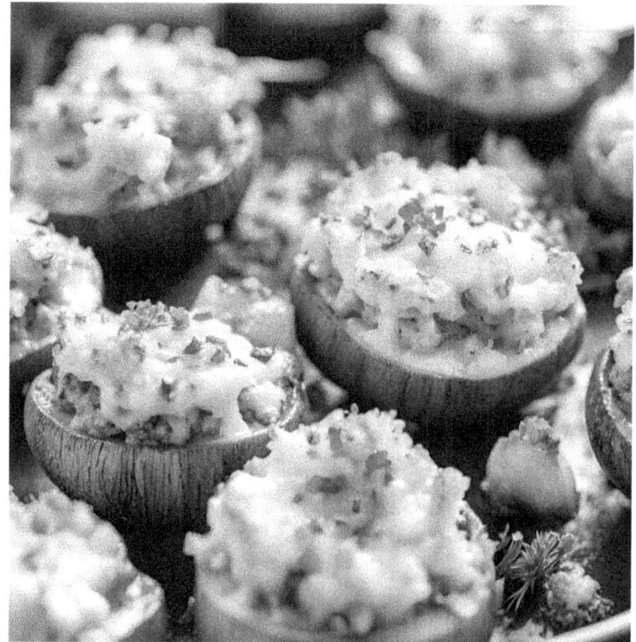

14. Ginger Soy Halibut

Ingredients

- 4 halibut fillets
- 1/4 cup low-sodium soy sauce
- 2 tablespoons olive oil
- 1 tablespoon grated fresh ginger
- 1/4 cup chopped green onions (green part only)
- Lemon wedges for serving

Instructions

1. Preheat the oven to 400°F (200°C).
2. In a small bowl, whisk together the soy sauce, olive oil, and grated ginger.
3. Place the halibut fillets in a baking dish and pour the soy sauce mixture over them, ensuring they are well coated.
4. Bake for 15-20 minutes, or until the fish is cooked through and flakes easily with a fork.
5. Garnish with chopped green onions and serve with lemon wedges.

Nutrition Information (Per Serving)

- Calories: 250
- Protein: 30g
- Carbohydrates: 2g
- Dietary Fiber: 0g
- Sugars: 0g
- Fat: 12g
- Saturated Fat: 2g
- Cholesterol: 70mg
- Sodium: 390mg

Servings

- **4 servings**

Cooking Time

- **25 minutes**

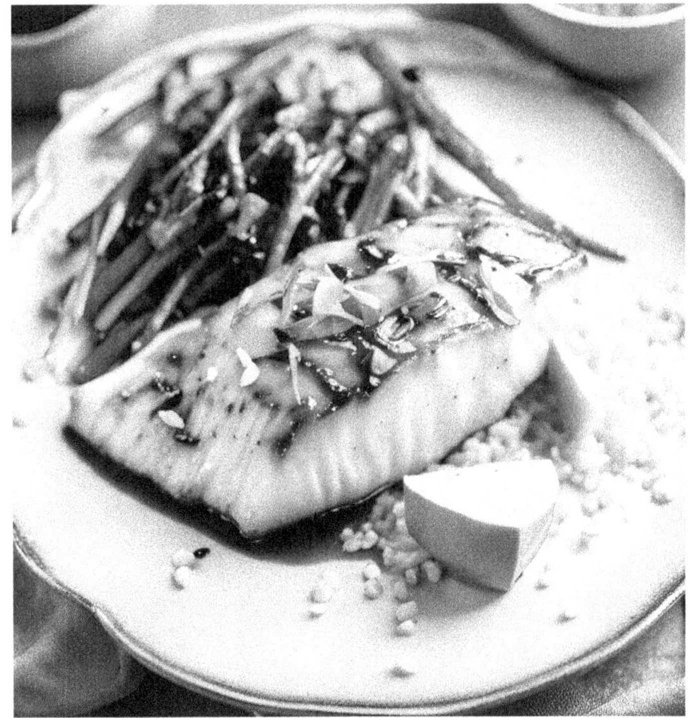

15. Steamed Sole with Ginger

Ingredients

- 4 sole fillets
- 2 tablespoons olive oil
- 1 tablespoon grated fresh ginger
- 1/4 cup low-sodium vegetable broth
- 1 tablespoon lemon juice
- 1/4 cup chopped green onions (green part only)
- Fresh cilantro for garnish (optional)

Instructions

1. Place the sole fillets in a steamer basket.
2. In a small bowl, whisk together the olive oil, grated ginger, vegetable broth, and lemon juice.
3. Pour the mixture over the sole fillets.
4. Steam the fish for 8-10 minutes, or until it is cooked through and flakes easily with a fork.
5. Garnish with chopped green onions and fresh cilantro if desired before serving.

Nutrition Information (Per Serving)

- Calories: 180
- Protein: 25g
- Carbohydrates: 2g
- Dietary Fiber: 0g
- Sugars: 0g
- Fat: 8g
- Saturated Fat: 1.5g
- Cholesterol: 70mg
- Sodium: 140mg

Servings

- **4 servings**

Cooking Time

- **15 minutes**

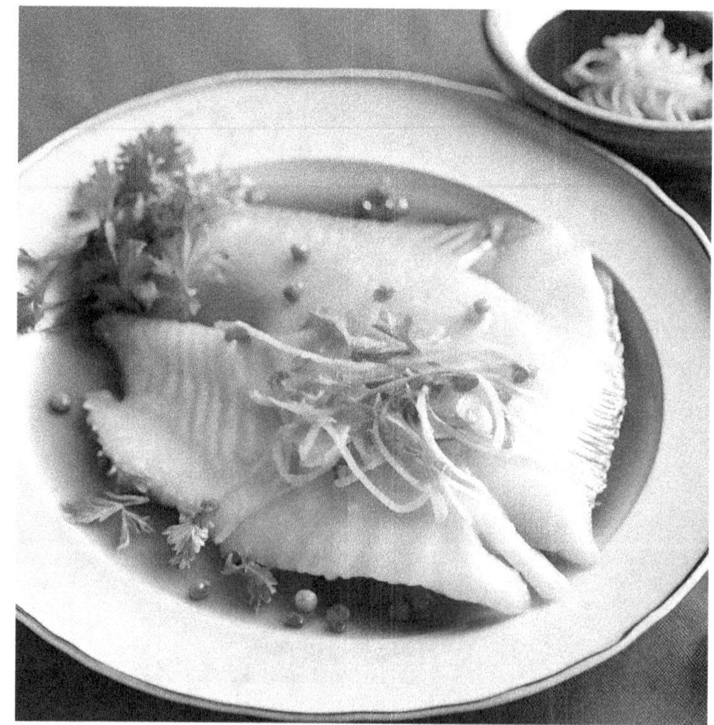

16. Salmon Burgers

Ingredients
- 1 pound skinless salmon fillets, finely chopped
- 1/2 cup whole wheat bread crumbs
- 1 large egg, beaten
- 1 tablespoon lemon juice
- 1 tablespoon chopped fresh dill
- 1/2 teaspoon ground paprika
- 1/4 teaspoon ground black pepper
- 2 tablespoons olive oil
- Whole grain burger buns
- Lettuce leaves (optional)
- Sliced avocado (optional)

Instructions
1. In a large bowl, combine the chopped salmon, whole wheat bread crumbs, beaten egg, lemon juice, chopped fresh dill, ground paprika, and ground black pepper. Mix until well combined.
2. Shape the mixture into 4 patties.
3. Heat the olive oil in a large skillet over medium heat.
4. Cook the salmon patties for 4-5 minutes on each side, until golden brown and cooked through.
5. Serve the salmon burgers on whole grain buns with lettuce leaves and sliced avocado if desired.

Nutrition Information (Per Serving)
- Calories: 350
- Protein: 28g
- Carbohydrates: 25g
- Dietary Fiber: 4g
- Sugars: 2g
- Fat: 15g
- Saturated Fat: 3g
- Cholesterol: 80mg
- Sodium: 250mg

Servings
- **4 servings**

Cooking Time
- **20 minutes**

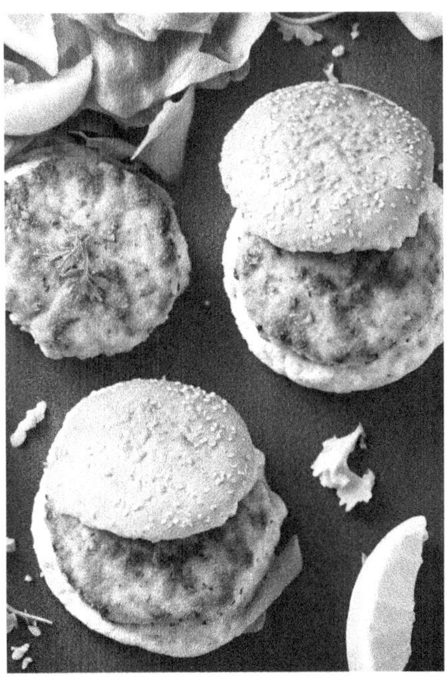

17. Panko-Crusted Cod

Ingredients

- 4 cod fillets
- 1/2 cup panko bread crumbs
- 1/4 cup grated Parmesan cheese
- 1 teaspoon dried oregano
- 1/2 teaspoon ground paprika
- 1/4 teaspoon ground black pepper
- 2 tablespoons olive oil
- Lemon wedges for serving

Instructions

1. Preheat the oven to 400°F (200°C) and line a baking sheet with parchment paper.
2. In a shallow dish, mix the panko bread crumbs, grated Parmesan cheese, dried oregano, ground paprika, and ground black pepper.
3. Brush each cod fillet with olive oil, then coat with the panko mixture, pressing lightly to adhere.
4. Place the coated fillets on the prepared baking sheet.
5. Bake for 12-15 minutes, or until the fish is golden brown and cooked through.
6. Serve with lemon wedges.

Nutrition Information (Per Serving)

- Calories: 300
- Protein: 30g
- Carbohydrates: 12g
- Dietary Fiber: 1g
- Sugars: 0g
- Fat: 15g
- Saturated Fat: 4g
- Cholesterol: 80mg
- Sodium: 300mg

Servings

- **4 servings**

Cooking Time

- **20 minutes**

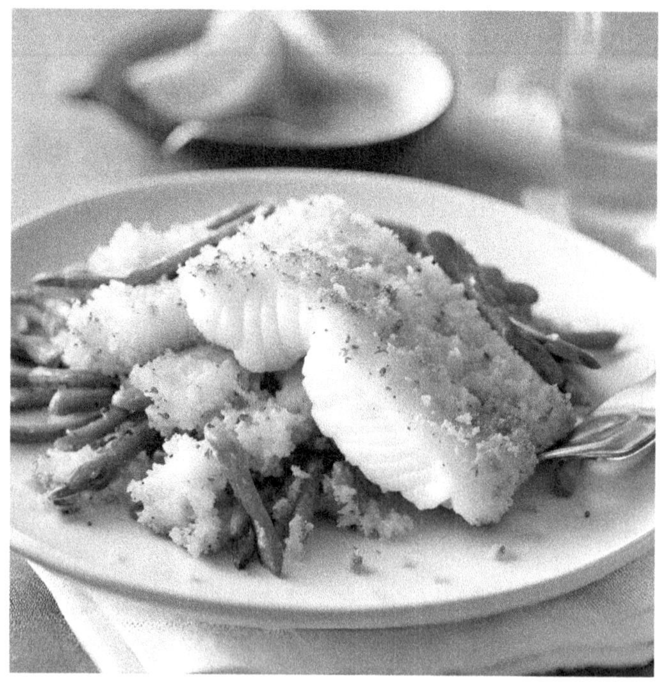

18. Halibut with Oat Crust

Ingredients

- 4 halibut fillets
- 1/2 cup rolled oats
- 1/4 cup whole wheat flour
- 1 teaspoon dried thyme
- 1/4 teaspoon ground black pepper
- 1 large egg, beaten
- 2 tablespoons olive oil

Instructions

1. Preheat the oven to 375°F (190°C) and line a baking sheet with parchment paper.
2. In a food processor, pulse the rolled oats until they resemble coarse breadcrumbs.
3. Set up a breading station with three shallow dishes: one with the whole wheat flour, one with the beaten egg, and one with the ground oats mixed with dried thyme and ground black pepper.
4. Dredge each halibut fillet in the flour, then dip in the egg, and finally coat with the oat mixture.
5. Heat the olive oil in a large skillet over medium heat.
6. Sear the halibut fillets for 2-3 minutes on each side, until golden brown.
7. Transfer the seared fillets to the prepared baking sheet and bake for 10-12 minutes, or until the fish is cooked through.
8. Serve immediately.

Nutrition Information (Per Serving)

- Calories: 320
- Protein: 32g
- Carbohydrates: 15g
- Dietary Fiber: 2g
- Sugars: 0g
- Fat: 14g
- Saturated Fat: 2.5g
- Cholesterol: 80mg
- Sodium: 200mg

Servings

- **4 servings**

Cooking Time

- **25 minutes**

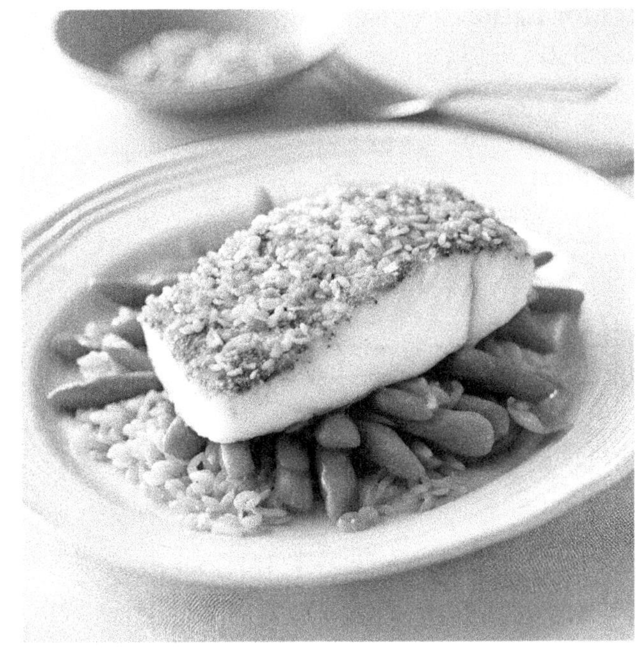

19. Shrimp and Rice Pilaf

Ingredients

- 1 cup basmati rice
- 2 cups low-sodium chicken broth
- 1 pound large shrimp, peeled and deveined
- 1/4 cup sliced almonds
- 1/4 cup raisins
- 1 tablespoon olive oil
- 1/2 teaspoon ground turmeric
- 1/4 teaspoon ground cumin
- 1/4 teaspoon ground cinnamon
- Fresh parsley for garnish (optional)

Instructions

1. In a medium saucepan, bring the chicken broth to a boil. Add the basmati rice, reduce the heat to low, cover, and simmer for 15 minutes, or until the rice is cooked and the liquid is absorbed.
2. In a large skillet, heat the olive oil over medium heat. Add the shrimp and cook for 2-3 minutes on each side, until pink and opaque. Remove from the skillet and set aside.
3. In the same skillet, add the sliced almonds and raisins. Cook for 2-3 minutes, until the almonds are toasted and the raisins are plump.
4. Add the cooked rice, ground turmeric, ground cumin, and ground cinnamon to the skillet. Stir to combine and cook for 2-3 minutes until heated through.
5. Return the shrimp to the skillet and stir gently to combine.
6. Garnish with fresh parsley before serving if desired.

Nutrition Information (Per Serving)

- Calories: 350
- Protein: 28g
- Carbohydrates: 40g
- Dietary Fiber: 3g
- Sugars: 6g
- Fat: 10g
- Saturated Fat: 1.5g
- Cholesterol: 190mg
- Sodium: 300mg

Servings

- **4 servings**

Cooking Time

- **25 minutes**

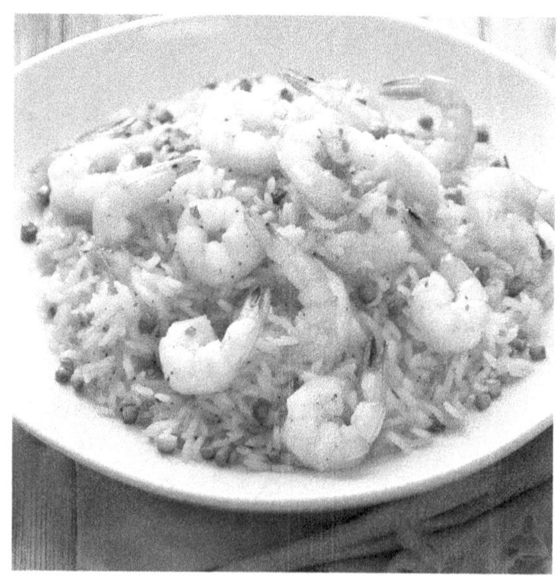

20. Herb-Crusted Trout

Ingredients

- 4 trout fillets
- 1/2 cup whole wheat bread crumbs
- 1/4 cup grated Parmesan cheese
- 2 tablespoons chopped fresh parsley
- 1 tablespoon chopped fresh dill
- 1 teaspoon dried thyme
- 2 tablespoons olive oil
- Lemon wedges for serving

Instructions

1. Preheat the oven to 375°F (190°C) and line a baking sheet with parchment paper.
2. In a bowl, mix the whole wheat bread crumbs, grated Parmesan cheese, chopped parsley, chopped dill, and dried thyme.
3. Brush each trout fillet with olive oil and then coat with the herb mixture, pressing lightly to adhere.
4. Place the coated fillets on the prepared baking sheet.
5. Bake for 15-20 minutes, or until the fish is golden brown and cooked through.
6. Serve with lemon wedges.

Nutrition Information (Per Serving)

- Calories: 250
- Protein: 28g
- Carbohydrates: 10g
- Dietary Fiber: 1g
- Sugars: 0g
- Fat: 12g
- Saturated Fat: 2g
- Cholesterol: 75mg
- Sodium: 250mg

Servings

- **4 servings**

Cooking Time

- **25 minutes**

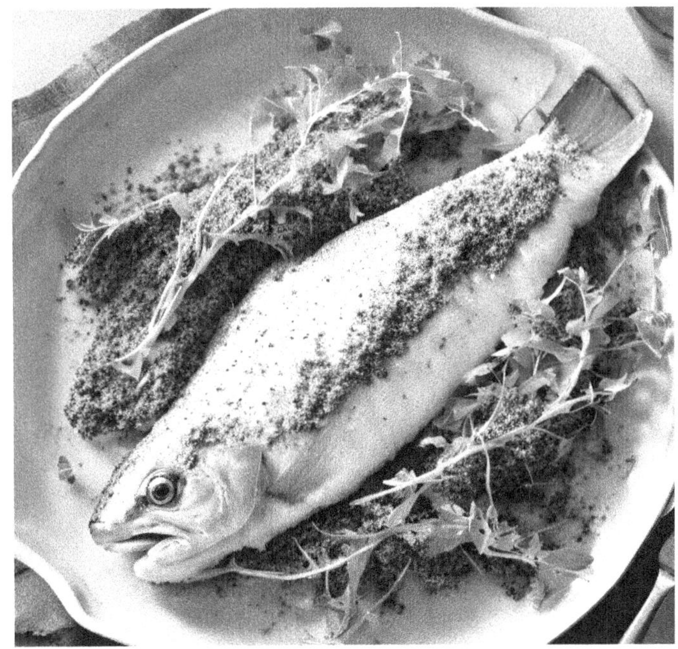

21. Salmon Chowder

Ingredients

- 1 pound salmon fillet, skin removed and cubed
- 2 cups low-sodium vegetable broth
- 1 cup diced potatoes
- 1 cup diced carrots
- 1 cup diced celery
- 1 cup corn kernels
- 1 cup almond milk (or any milk of your choice)
- 1 tablespoon olive oil
- 1 teaspoon dried thyme
- 1/2 teaspoon ground black pepper
- 1/4 cup chopped fresh parsley

Instructions

1. In a large pot, heat the olive oil over medium heat.
2. Add the diced potatoes, carrots, and celery. Cook for 5-7 minutes, stirring occasionally, until the vegetables begin to soften.
3. Add the vegetable broth, corn kernels, dried thyme, and ground black pepper. Bring to a boil, then reduce the heat and simmer for 15 minutes.
4. Stir in the almond milk and cubed salmon. Cook for an additional 5-7 minutes, or until the salmon is cooked through.
5. Garnish with fresh parsley before serving.

Nutrition Information (Per Serving)

- Calories: 300
- Protein: 25g
- Carbohydrates: 25g
- Dietary Fiber: 4g
- Sugars: 5g
- Fat: 12g
- Saturated Fat: 2g
- Cholesterol: 60mg
- Sodium: 250mg

Servings

- **4 servings**

Cooking Time

- **30 minutes**

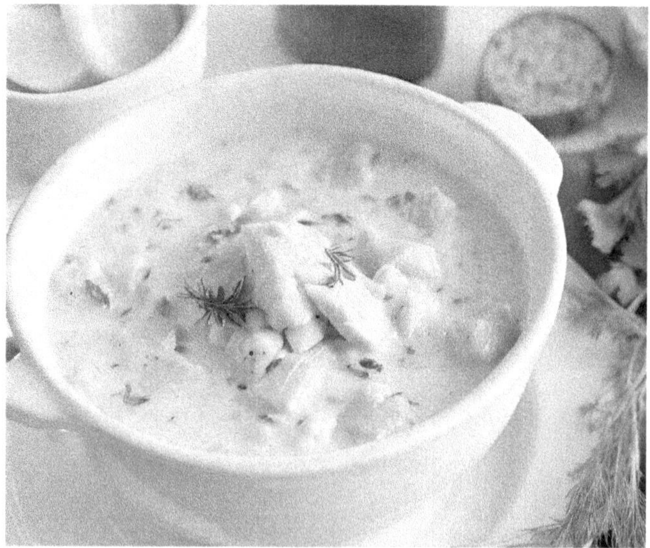

22. Scallops with Basil

Ingredients

- 1 pound sea scallops
- 2 tablespoons olive oil
- 1/4 cup low-sodium vegetable broth
- 1 tablespoon lemon juice
- 1/4 cup chopped fresh basil
- 1/2 teaspoon ground paprika
- Fresh basil leaves for garnish (optional)

Instructions

1. Pat the scallops dry with paper towels.
2. In a large skillet, heat the olive oil over medium-high heat.
3. Add the scallops and cook for 2-3 minutes on each side, until they are golden brown and cooked through. Remove from the skillet and keep warm.
4. In the same skillet, add the vegetable broth, lemon juice, and ground paprika. Cook for 2-3 minutes, stirring occasionally, until the sauce is slightly reduced.
5. Stir in the chopped basil.
6. Return the scallops to the skillet and toss gently to coat with the sauce.
7. Serve immediately, garnished with fresh basil leaves if desired.

Nutrition Information (Per Serving)

- Calories: 220
- Protein: 24g
- Carbohydrates: 3g
- Dietary Fiber: 0g
- Sugars: 0g
- Fat: 12g
- Saturated Fat: 2g
- Cholesterol: 40mg
- Sodium: 270mg

Servings

- **4 servings**

Cooking Time

- **15 minutes**

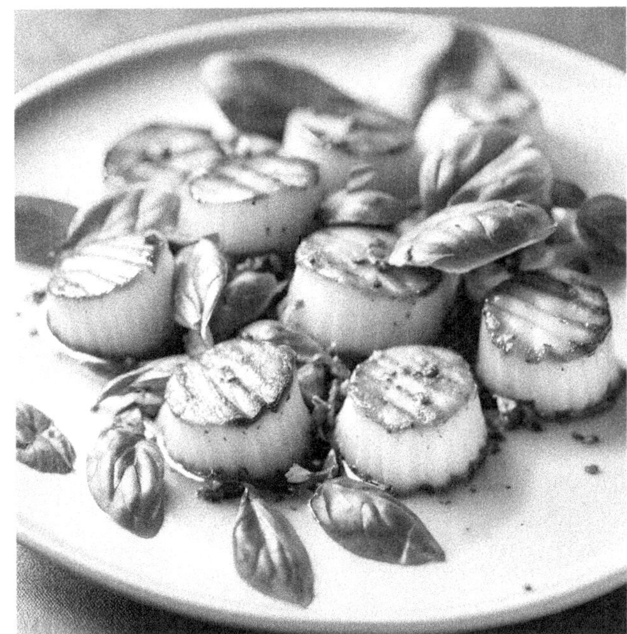

23. Flounder with Spinach

Ingredients

- 4 flounder fillets
- 2 tablespoons olive oil
- 1/4 cup low-sodium vegetable broth
- 1 tablespoon lemon juice
- 1/4 teaspoon ground black pepper
- 4 cups fresh spinach
- Lemon wedges for serving

Instructions

1. Preheat the oven to 375°F (190°C) and line a baking sheet with parchment paper.
2. Place the flounder fillets on the prepared baking sheet.
3. In a small bowl, mix the olive oil, vegetable broth, lemon juice, and ground black pepper. Drizzle the mixture over the flounder fillets.
4. Bake for 12-15 minutes, or until the fish is cooked through and flakes easily with a fork.
5. While the fish is baking, heat a large skillet over medium heat. Add the fresh spinach and cook for 2-3 minutes, until wilted.
6. Serve the flounder fillets over the wilted spinach, with lemon wedges on the side.

Nutrition Information (Per Serving)

- Calories: 200
- Protein: 25g
- Carbohydrates: 4g
- Dietary Fiber: 2g
- Sugars: 0g
- Fat: 10g
- Saturated Fat: 1.5g
- Cholesterol: 70mg
- Sodium: 180mg

Servings

- **4 servings**

Cooking Time

- **20 minutes**

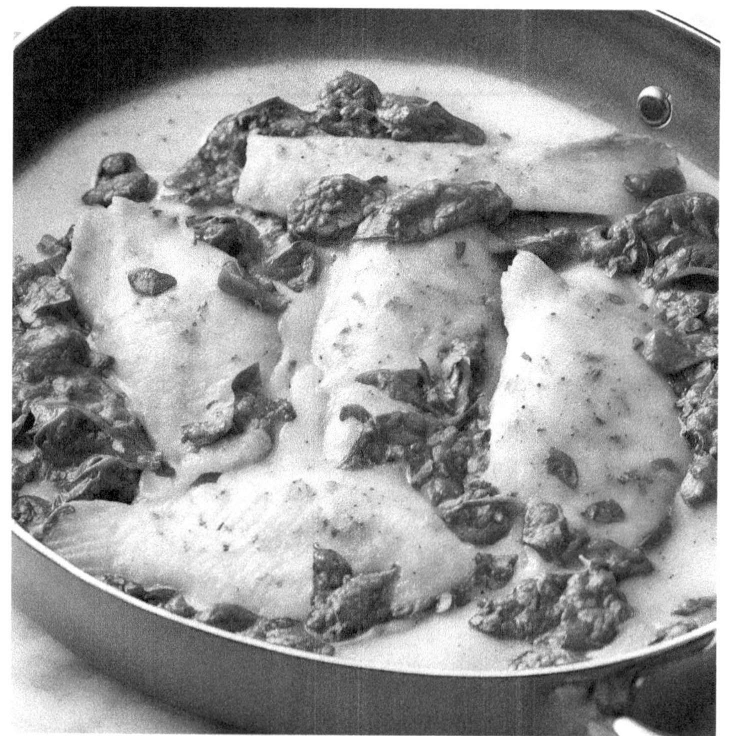

24. Sea Bass with Parsley Sauce

Ingredients

- 4 sea bass fillets
- 2 tablespoons olive oil
- 1/2 cup low-sodium vegetable broth
- 1/4 cup chopped fresh parsley
- 1 tablespoon lemon juice
- 1/2 teaspoon ground paprika
- Lemon wedges for serving

Instructions

1. Preheat the oven to 375°F (190°C) and line a baking sheet with parchment paper.
2. Brush the sea bass fillets with olive oil and place them on the prepared baking sheet.
3. In a small bowl, mix the vegetable broth, chopped parsley, lemon juice, and ground paprika.
4. Pour the parsley sauce over the sea bass fillets.
5. Bake for 15-20 minutes, or until the fish is cooked through and flakes easily with a fork.
6. Serve with lemon wedges.

Nutrition Information (Per Serving)

- Calories: 240
- Protein: 28g
- Carbohydrates: 3g
- Dietary Fiber: 1g
- Sugars: 0g
- Fat: 12g
- Saturated Fat: 2g
- Cholesterol: 70mg
- Sodium: 200mg

Servings

- **4 servings**

Cooking Time

- **25 minutes**

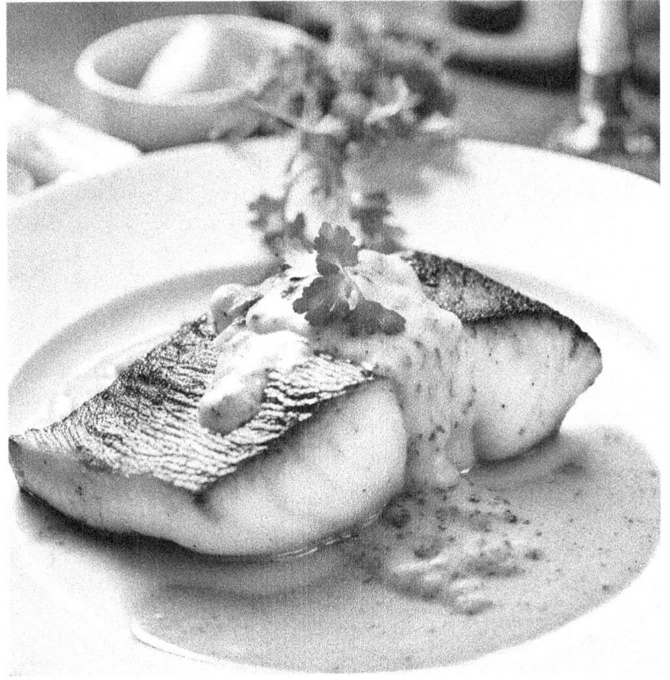

25. Grilled Shrimp Skewers

Ingredients

- 1 pound large shrimp, peeled and deveined
- 2 tablespoons olive oil
- 1 tablespoon lemon juice
- 1 teaspoon dried oregano
- 1/2 teaspoon ground paprika
- Wooden or metal skewers
- Lemon wedges for serving

Instructions

1. In a large bowl, mix the olive oil, lemon juice, dried oregano, and ground paprika.
2. Add the shrimp to the bowl and toss to coat evenly. Let marinate for 15 minutes.
3. Preheat the grill to medium-high heat.
4. Thread the shrimp onto skewers.
5. Grill the shrimp skewers for 2-3 minutes on each side, until the shrimp are pink and opaque.
6. Serve with lemon wedges.

Nutrition Information (Per Serving)

- Calories: 220
- Protein: 26g
- Carbohydrates: 2g
- Dietary Fiber: 0g
- Sugars: 0g
- Fat: 12g
- Saturated Fat: 2g
- Cholesterol: 190mg
- Sodium: 340mg

Servings

- **4 servings**

Cooking Time

- **20 minutes**

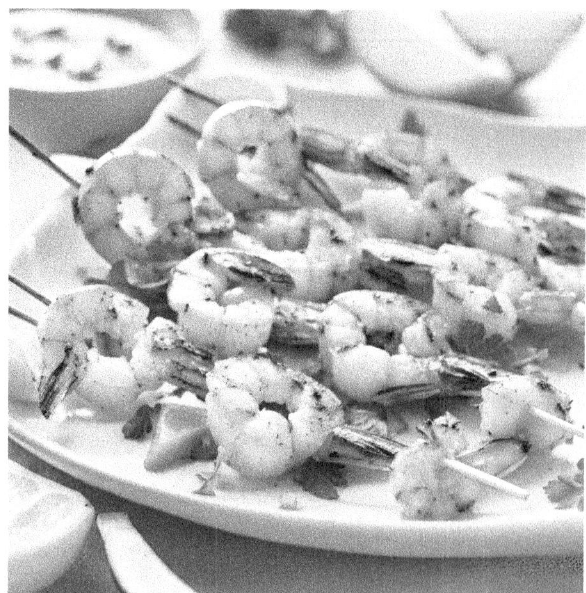

26. Tilapia with Mango Salsa

Ingredients

- 4 tilapia fillets
- 2 tablespoons olive oil
- 1 tablespoon lemon juice
- 1 teaspoon ground cumin
- 1 ripe mango, peeled, pitted, and diced
- 1/2 cup diced cucumber
- 1/4 cup chopped fresh cilantro
- 1 tablespoon lime juice

Instructions

1. Preheat the oven to 375°F (190°C) and line a baking sheet with parchment paper.
2. Brush the tilapia fillets with olive oil and drizzle with lemon juice. Sprinkle with ground cumin.
3. Bake for 12-15 minutes, or until the fish is cooked through and flakes easily with a fork.
4. While the fish is baking, prepare the mango salsa by combining the diced mango, diced cucumber, chopped cilantro, and lime juice in a bowl.
5. Serve the tilapia topped with mango salsa.

Nutrition Information (Per Serving)

- Calories: 240
- Protein: 25g
- Carbohydrates: 10g
- Dietary Fiber: 2g
- Sugars: 6g
- Fat: 12g
- Saturated Fat: 2g
- Cholesterol: 70mg
- Sodium: 150mg

Servings

- 4 servings

Cooking Time

- 20 minutes

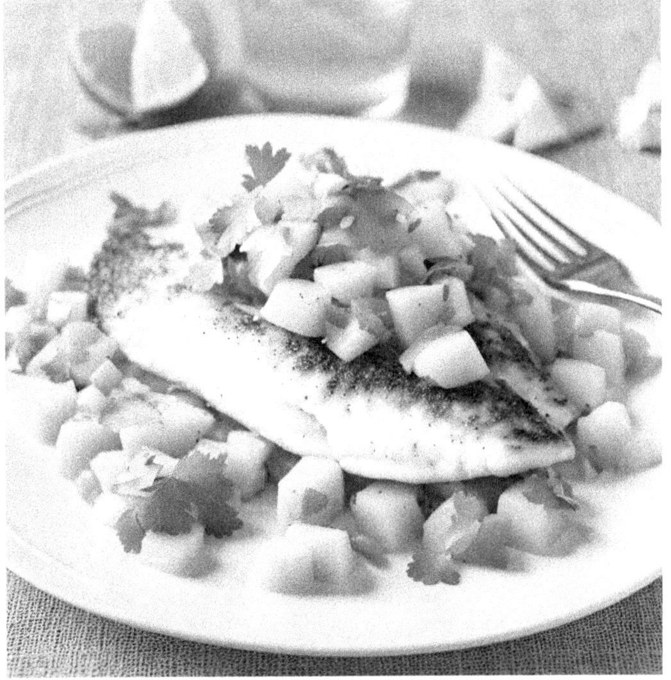

27. Poached Salmon

Ingredients

- 4 salmon fillets
- 4 cups low-sodium vegetable broth
- 1/2 cup lemon juice
- 2 tablespoons fresh dill, chopped
- 1 teaspoon ground black pepper
- Lemon wedges for serving

Instructions

1. In a large skillet, bring the vegetable broth, lemon juice, fresh dill, and ground black pepper to a gentle simmer.
2. Add the salmon fillets to the skillet, ensuring they are fully submerged in the liquid.
3. Cover and poach the salmon for 8-10 minutes, or until the fish is opaque and flakes easily with a fork.
4. Carefully remove the salmon from the skillet and serve with lemon wedges.

Nutrition Information (Per Serving)

- Calories: 280
- Protein: 28g
- Carbohydrates: 3g
- Dietary Fiber: 0g
- Sugars: 1g
- Fat: 16g
- Saturated Fat: 3g
- Cholesterol: 80mg
- Sodium: 200mg

Servings

- **4 servings**

Cooking Time

- **15 minutes**

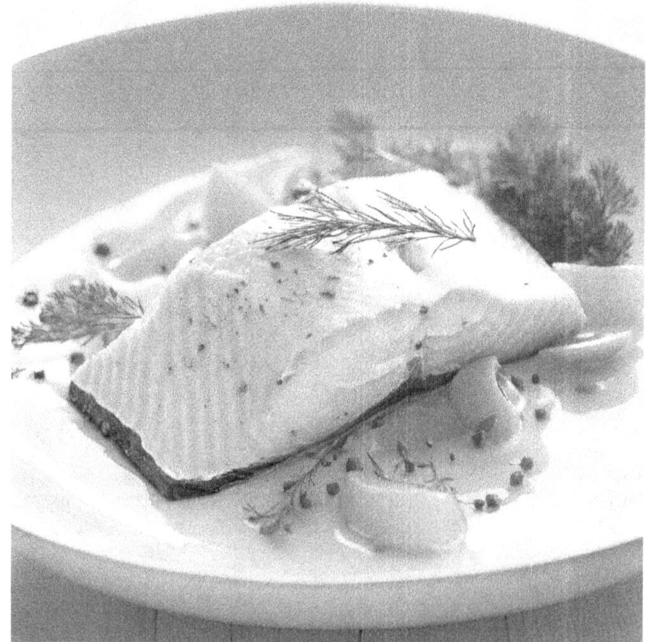

Vegetables

1. Steamed Broccoli with Olive Oil

Ingredients

- 4 cups broccoli florets
- 2 tablespoons olive oil
- 1 teaspoon lemon juice
- 1/2 teaspoon ground black pepper

Instructions

1. Bring a pot of water to a boil and place a steamer basket over it.
2. Add the broccoli florets to the steamer basket and cover. Steam for 5-7 minutes, or until the broccoli is tender.
3. Transfer the steamed broccoli to a serving bowl.
4. Drizzle with olive oil and lemon juice.
5. Sprinkle with ground black pepper and toss to combine.
6. Serve immediately.

Nutrition Information (Per Serving)

- Calories: 100
- Protein: 3g
- Carbohydrates: 7g
- Dietary Fiber: 3g
- Sugars: 2g
- Fat: 7g
- Saturated Fat: 1g
- Cholesterol: 0mg
- Sodium: 40mg

Servings

- **4 servings**

Cooking Time

- **10 minutes**

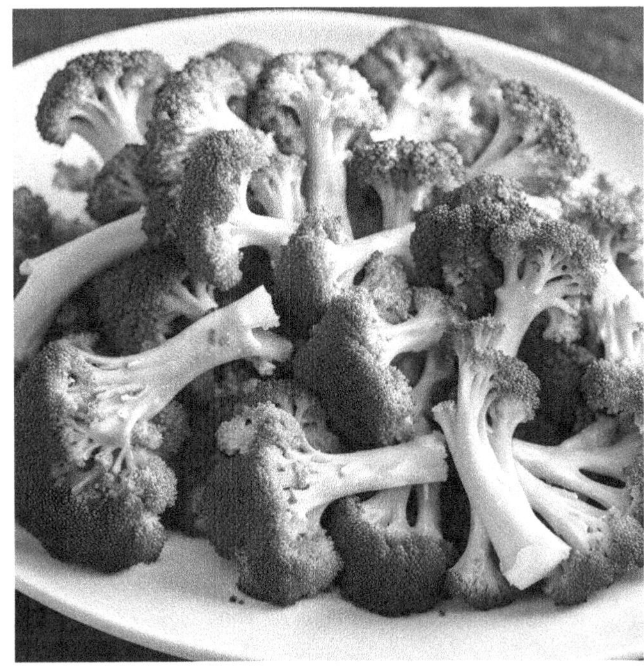

2. Baked Butternut Squash

Ingredients

- 1 medium butternut squash, peeled, seeded, and cubed
- 2 tablespoons olive oil
- 1 teaspoon ground cinnamon
- 1/2 teaspoon ground nutmeg
- 1 tablespoon honey

Instructions

1. Preheat the oven to 400°F (200°C) and line a baking sheet with parchment paper.
2. In a large bowl, toss the butternut squash cubes with olive oil, ground cinnamon, ground nutmeg, and honey.
3. Spread the squash evenly on the prepared baking sheet.
4. Bake for 25-30 minutes, or until the squash is tender and lightly browned, stirring halfway through.
5. Serve warm.

Nutrition Information (Per Serving)

- Calories: 120
- Protein: 1g
- Carbohydrates: 16g
- Dietary Fiber: 3g
- Sugars: 7g
- Fat: 7g
- Saturated Fat: 1g
- Cholesterol: 0mg
- Sodium: 20mg

Servings

- **4 servings**

Cooking Time

- **35 minutes**

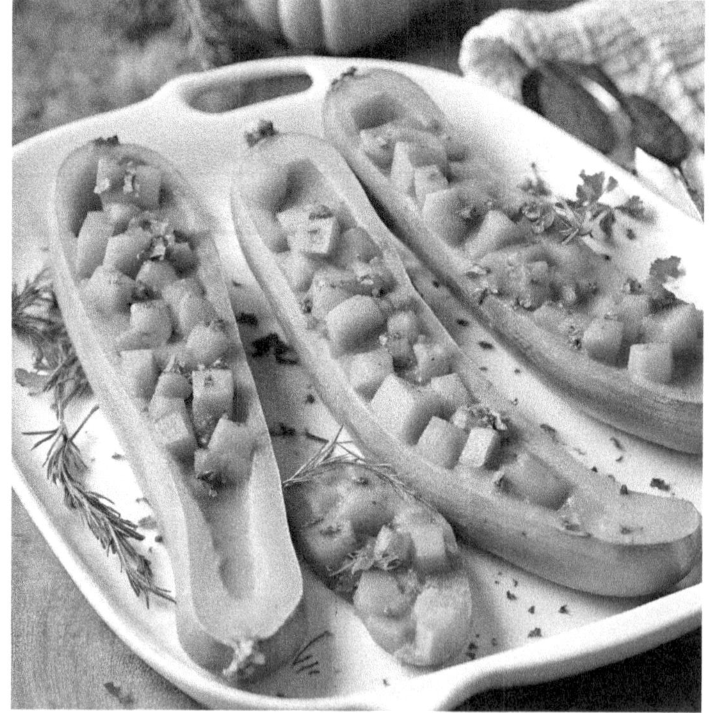

3. Carrot and Zucchini Ribbons

Ingredients

- 2 large carrots
- 2 medium zucchinis
- 2 tablespoons olive oil
- 1 tablespoon lemon juice
- 1/2 teaspoon dried oregano
- 1/4 teaspoon ground black pepper

Instructions

1. Using a vegetable peeler, peel the carrots and zucchinis into long, thin ribbons.
2. In a large skillet, heat the olive oil over medium heat.
3. Add the carrot and zucchini ribbons to the skillet and sauté for 3-5 minutes, or until just tender.
4. Remove from heat and drizzle with lemon juice.
5. Sprinkle with dried oregano and ground black pepper, and toss to combine.
6. Serve immediately.

Nutrition Information (Per Serving)

- Calories: 80
- Protein: 1g
- Carbohydrates: 7g
- Dietary Fiber: 2g
- Sugars: 4g
- Fat: 7g
- Saturated Fat: 1g
- Cholesterol: 0mg
- Sodium: 10mg

Servings

- **4 servings**

Cooking Time

- **10 minutes**

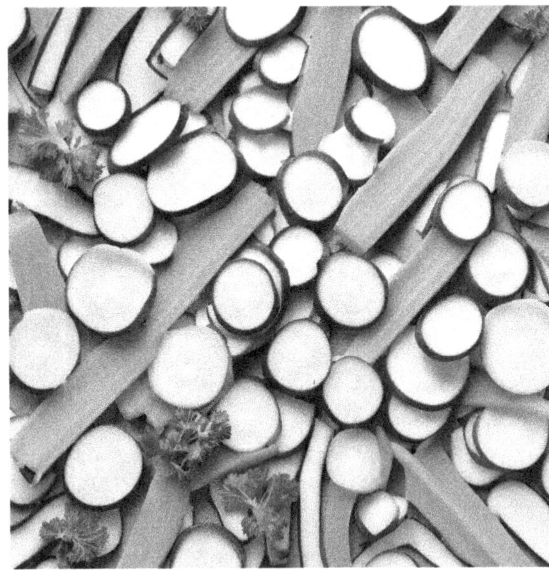

4. Sauteed Spinach with Pine Nuts

Ingredients

- 6 cups fresh spinach leaves
- 2 tablespoons olive oil
- 1/4 cup pine nuts
- 1/4 teaspoon ground black pepper

Instructions

1. In a large skillet, heat the olive oil over medium heat.
2. Add the pine nuts and cook, stirring frequently, for 2-3 minutes, or until they are lightly toasted.
3. Add the spinach to the skillet and sauté for 2-3 minutes, or until the spinach is wilted.
4. Sprinkle with ground black pepper and toss to combine.
5. Serve immediately.

Nutrition Information (Per Serving)

- Calories: 120
- Protein: 3g
- Carbohydrates: 4g
- Dietary Fiber: 2g
- Sugars: 1g
- Fat: 11g
- Saturated Fat: 1.5g
- Cholesterol: 0mg
- Sodium: 45mg

Servings

- **4 servings**

Cooking Time

- **10 minutes**

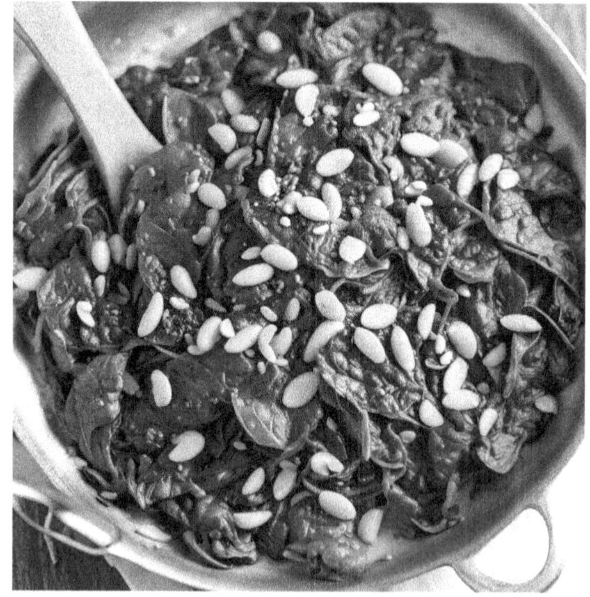

5. Roasted Beets with Thyme

Ingredients

- 4 medium beets, peeled and cut into wedges
- 2 tablespoons olive oil
- 1 tablespoon fresh thyme leaves
- 1 tablespoon honey

Instructions

1. Preheat the oven to 400°F (200°C) and line a baking sheet with parchment paper.
2. In a large bowl, toss the beet wedges with olive oil, fresh thyme leaves, and honey.
3. Spread the beets evenly on the prepared baking sheet.
4. Roast for 30-35 minutes, or until the beets are tender and caramelized, stirring halfway through.
5. Serve warm.

Nutrition Information (Per Serving)

- Calories: 110
- Protein: 2g
- Carbohydrates: 15g
- Dietary Fiber: 4g
- Sugars: 9g
- Fat: 6g
- Saturated Fat: 1g
- Cholesterol: 0mg
- Sodium: 70mg

Servings

- **4 servings**

Cooking Time

- **40 minutes**

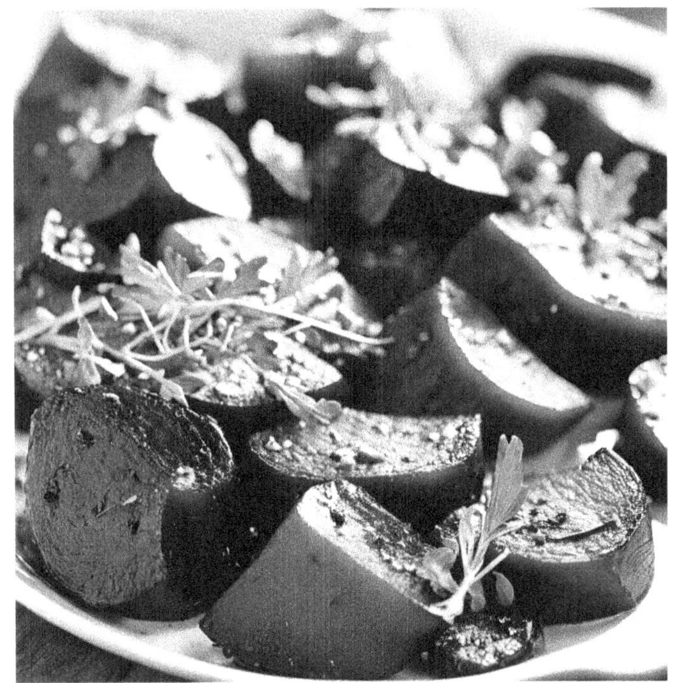

6. Creamy Parsnip Soup

Ingredients

- 4 large parsnips, peeled and chopped
- 1 medium potato, peeled and chopped
- 4 cups low-sodium vegetable broth
- 1 cup unsweetened almond milk
- 2 tablespoons olive oil
- 1 teaspoon dried thyme
- 1/2 teaspoon ground black pepper

Instructions

1. In a large pot, heat the olive oil over medium heat.
2. Add the chopped parsnips and potato, and sauté for 5-7 minutes until they begin to soften.
3. Add the vegetable broth and dried thyme. Bring to a boil, then reduce the heat and simmer for 20-25 minutes, or until the vegetables are tender.
4. Use an immersion blender to puree the soup until smooth (or transfer to a blender in batches if you do not have an immersion blender).
5. Stir in the almond milk and ground black pepper, and heat through.
6. Serve warm.

Nutrition Information (Per Serving)

- Calories: 180
- Protein: 3g
- Carbohydrates: 30g
- Dietary Fiber: 6g
- Sugars: 8g
- Fat: 7g
- Saturated Fat: 1g
- Cholesterol: 0mg
- Sodium: 150mg

Servings

- **4 servings**

Cooking Time

- **35 minutes**

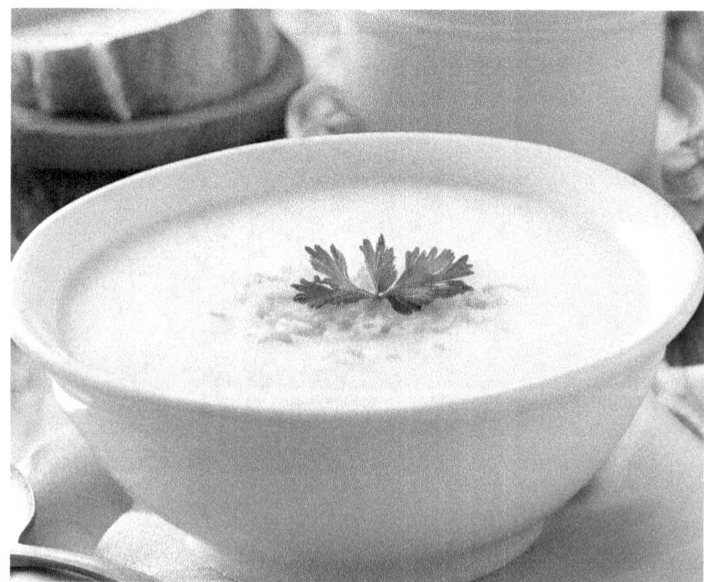

7. Steamed Green Beans

Ingredients

- 1 pound fresh green beans, trimmed
- 2 tablespoons olive oil
- 1 tablespoon lemon juice
- 1/4 teaspoon ground black pepper

Instructions

1. Bring a pot of water to a boil and place a steamer basket over it.
2. Add the green beans to the steamer basket and cover. Steam for 5-7 minutes, or until the green beans are tender.
3. Transfer the steamed green beans to a serving bowl.
4. Drizzle with olive oil and lemon juice.
5. Sprinkle with ground black pepper and toss to combine.
6. Serve immediately.

Nutrition Information (Per Serving)

- Calories: 90
- Protein: 2g
- Carbohydrates: 8g
- Dietary Fiber: 3g
- Sugars: 4g
- Fat: 7g
- Saturated Fat: 1g
- Cholesterol: 0mg
- Sodium: 15mg

Servings

- **4 servings**

Cooking Time

- **10 minutes**

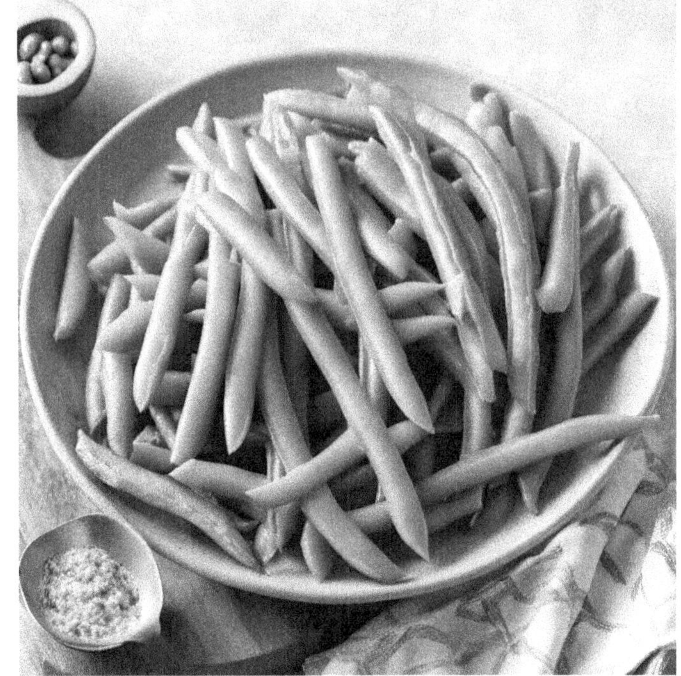

8. Cauliflower Puree

Ingredients

- 1 large head cauliflower, cut into florets
- 1 cup low-sodium vegetable broth
- 1/2 cup unsweetened almond milk
- 2 tablespoons olive oil
- 1/2 teaspoon ground nutmeg

Instructions

1. Bring a large pot of water to a boil. Add the cauliflower florets and cook for 10-12 minutes, or until very tender.
2. Drain the cauliflower and transfer to a blender or food processor.
3. Add the vegetable broth, almond milk, olive oil, and ground nutmeg.
4. Blend until smooth and creamy.
5. Serve warm.

Nutrition Information (Per Serving)

- Calories: 100
- Protein: 3g
- Carbohydrates: 10g
- Dietary Fiber: 4g
- Sugars: 3g
- Fat: 7g
- Saturated Fat: 1g
- Cholesterol: 0mg
- Sodium: 60mg

Servings

- **4 servings**

Cooking Time

- **15 minutes**

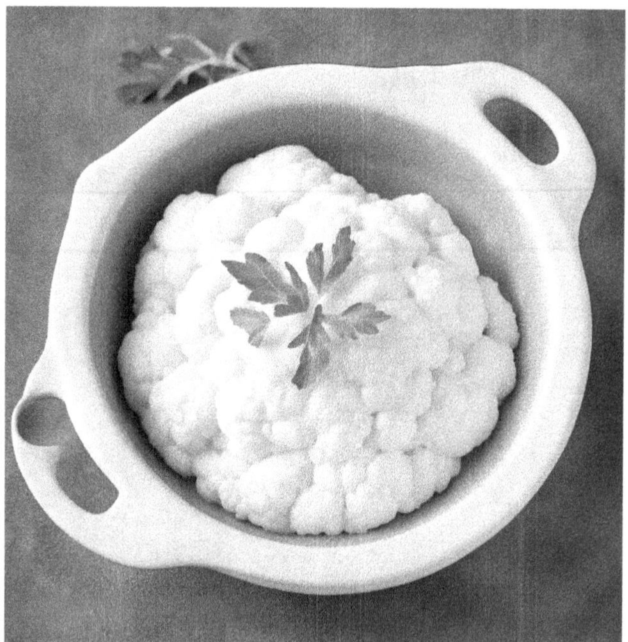

9. Roasted Root Vegetables

Ingredients

- 2 medium carrots, peeled and chopped
- 2 medium parsnips, peeled and chopped
- 2 medium sweet potatoes, peeled and chopped
- 2 tablespoons olive oil
- 1 teaspoon dried rosemary
- 1/2 teaspoon ground black pepper

Instructions

1. Preheat the oven to 400°F (200°C) and line a baking sheet with parchment paper.
2. In a large bowl, toss the chopped carrots, parsnips, and sweet potatoes with olive oil, dried rosemary, and ground black pepper.
3. Spread the vegetables evenly on the prepared baking sheet.
4. Roast for 25-30 minutes, or until the vegetables are tender and lightly browned, stirring halfway through.
5. Serve warm.

Nutrition Information (Per Serving)

- Calories: 140
- Protein: 2g
- Carbohydrates: 24g
- Dietary Fiber: 5g
- Sugars: 7g
- Fat: 6g
- Saturated Fat: 1g
- Cholesterol: 0mg
- Sodium: 55mg

Servings

- **4 servings**

Cooking Time

- **35 minutes**

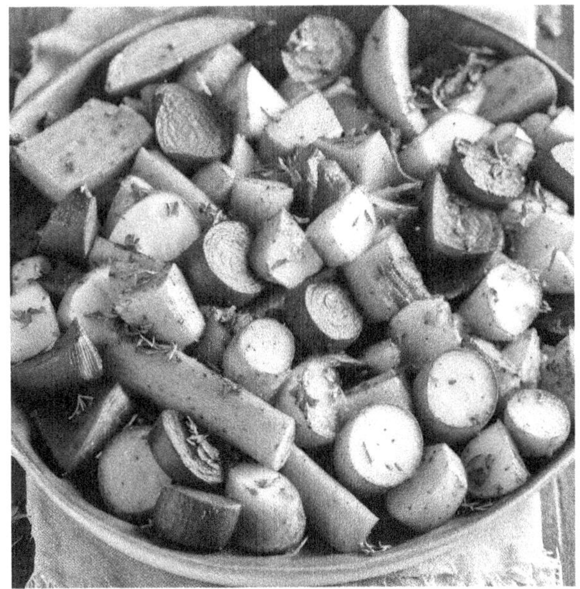

10. Baked Parsnip Fries

Ingredients

- 4 large parsnips, peeled and cut into fries
- 2 tablespoons olive oil
- 1 teaspoon dried thyme
- 1/4 teaspoon ground black pepper

Instructions

1. Preheat the oven to 400°F (200°C) and line a baking sheet with parchment paper.
2. In a large bowl, toss the parsnip fries with olive oil, dried thyme, and ground black pepper.
3. Spread the parsnip fries evenly on the prepared baking sheet.
4. Bake for 25-30 minutes, or until the fries are golden brown and crispy, turning halfway through.
5. Serve warm.

Nutrition Information (Per Serving)

- Calories: 120
- Protein: 2g
- Carbohydrates: 20g
- Dietary Fiber: 5g
- Sugars: 6g
- Fat: 6g
- Saturated Fat: 1g
- Cholesterol: 0mg
- Sodium: 30mg

Servings

- **4 servings**

Cooking Time

- **35 minutes**

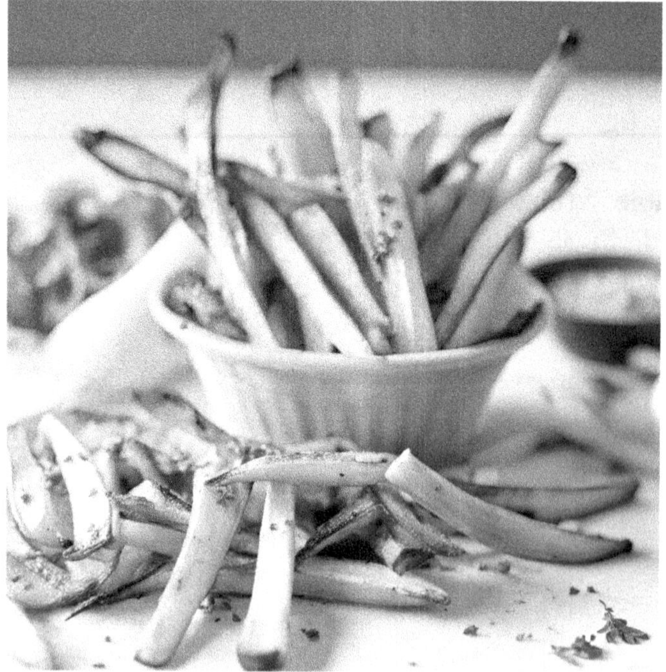

11. Stuffed Mushrooms

Ingredients

- 1 pound large white mushrooms, stems removed
- 1 cup cooked quinoa
- 1/4 cup plain Greek yogurt
- 1/4 cup grated Parmesan cheese (optional)
- 2 tablespoons chopped fresh parsley
- 1 teaspoon dried oregano
- 1/4 teaspoon ground black pepper

Instructions

1. Preheat the oven to 375°F (190°C) and line a baking sheet with parchment paper.
2. In a bowl, mix the cooked quinoa, Greek yogurt, grated Parmesan cheese (if using), chopped parsley, dried oregano, and ground black pepper.
3. Stuff each mushroom cap with the quinoa mixture and place them on the prepared baking sheet.
4. Bake for 15-20 minutes, or until the mushrooms are tender and the filling is golden brown.
5. Serve warm.

Nutrition Information (Per Serving)

- Calories: 100
- Protein: 6g
- Carbohydrates: 10g
- Dietary Fiber: 2g
- Sugars: 2g
- Fat: 4g
- Saturated Fat: 1.5g
- Cholesterol: 10mg
- Sodium: 80mg

Servings

- **4 servings**

Cooking Time

- **25 minutes**

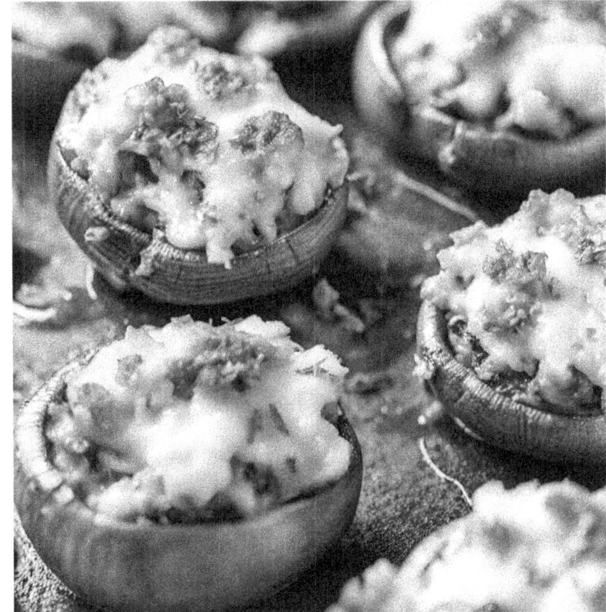

12. Brussels Sprouts with Chestnuts

Ingredients

- 4 cups Brussels sprouts, trimmed and halved
- 1 cup cooked chestnuts, halved
- 2 tablespoons olive oil
- 1/4 teaspoon ground black pepper

Instructions

1. Preheat the oven to 400°F (200°C) and line a baking sheet with parchment paper.
2. In a large bowl, toss the Brussels sprouts and chestnuts with olive oil and ground black pepper.
3. Spread the Brussels sprouts and chestnuts evenly on the prepared baking sheet.
4. Roast for 20-25 minutes, or until the Brussels sprouts are tender and lightly browned.
5. Serve warm.

Nutrition Information (Per Serving)

- Calories: 150
- Protein: 4g
- Carbohydrates: 22g
- Dietary Fiber: 7g
- Sugars: 4g
- Fat: 7g
- Saturated Fat: 1g
- Cholesterol: 0mg
- Sodium: 50mg

Servings

- **4 servings**

Cooking Time

- **30 minutes**

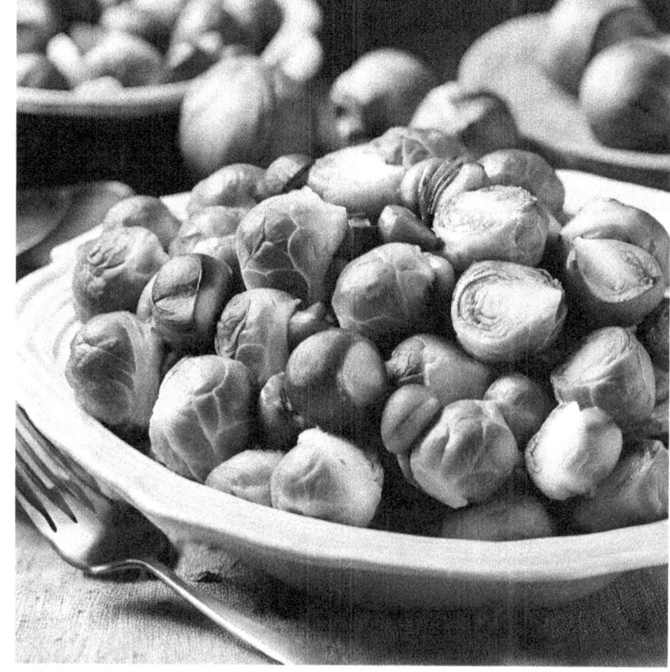

13. Creamy Carrot Soup

Ingredients

- 1 pound carrots, peeled and chopped
- 1 medium potato, peeled and chopped
- 4 cups low-sodium vegetable broth
- 1 cup unsweetened almond milk
- 2 tablespoons olive oil
- 1 teaspoon dried thyme
- 1/4 teaspoon ground black pepper

Instructions

1. In a large pot, heat the olive oil over medium heat.
2. Add the chopped carrots and potato, and sauté for 5-7 minutes until they begin to soften.
3. Add the vegetable broth and dried thyme. Bring to a boil, then reduce the heat and simmer for 20-25 minutes, or until the vegetables are tender.
4. Use an immersion blender to puree the soup until smooth (or transfer to a blender in batches if you do not have an immersion blender).
5. Stir in the almond milk and ground black pepper, and heat through.
6. Serve warm.

Nutrition Information (Per Serving)

- Calories: 160
- Protein: 3g
- Carbohydrates: 24g
- Dietary Fiber: 5g
- Sugars: 10g
- Fat: 7g
- Saturated Fat: 1g
- Cholesterol: 0mg
- Sodium: 160mg

Servings

- **4 servings**

Cooking Time

- **35 minutes**

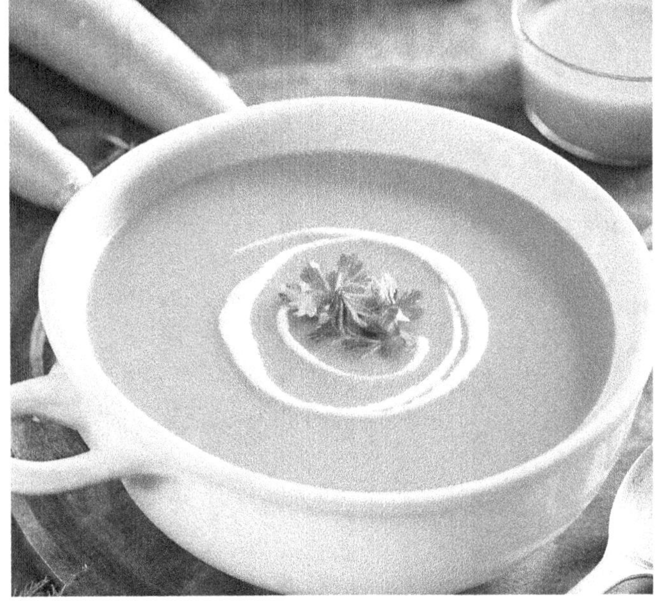

14. Celery Root Mash

Ingredients

- 1 large celery root, peeled and chopped
- 2 medium potatoes, peeled and chopped
- 4 cups low-sodium vegetable broth
- 1/2 cup unsweetened almond milk
- 2 tablespoons olive oil
- 1/4 teaspoon ground nutmeg

Instructions

1. In a large pot, bring the vegetable broth to a boil.
2. Add the chopped celery root and potatoes. Reduce the heat and simmer for 20-25 minutes, or until the vegetables are tender.
3. Drain the vegetables and return them to the pot.
4. Add the almond milk, olive oil, and ground nutmeg.
5. Mash until smooth and creamy.
6. Serve warm.

Nutrition Information (Per Serving)

- Calories: 130
- Protein: 2g
- Carbohydrates: 20g
- Dietary Fiber: 4g
- Sugars: 3g
- Fat: 6g
- Saturated Fat: 1g
- Cholesterol: 0mg
- Sodium: 80mg

Servings

- **4 servings**

Cooking Time

- **30 minutes**

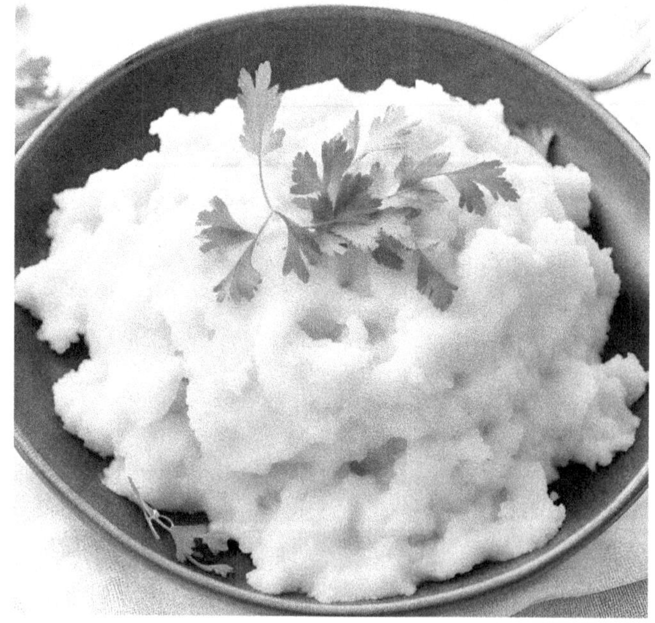

15. Baked Leeks

Ingredients

- 4 large leeks, white and light green parts only, halved lengthwise and cleaned
- 2 tablespoons olive oil
- 1 teaspoon dried thyme
- 1/4 teaspoon ground black pepper
- 1/4 cup grated Parmesan cheese (optional)

Instructions

1. Preheat the oven to 375°F (190°C) and line a baking dish with parchment paper.
2. Place the halved leeks in the prepared baking dish.
3. Drizzle with olive oil and sprinkle with dried thyme and ground black pepper.
4. Cover the dish with aluminum foil and bake for 25-30 minutes, or until the leeks are tender.
5. If using, sprinkle with grated Parmesan cheese and bake uncovered for an additional 5 minutes.
6. Serve warm.

Nutrition Information (Per Serving)

- Calories: 110
- Protein: 2g
- Carbohydrates: 12g
- Dietary Fiber: 3g
- Sugars: 4g
- Fat: 6g
- Saturated Fat: 1g
- Cholesterol: 0mg
- Sodium: 60mg

Servings

- **4 servings**

Cooking Time

- **35 minutes**

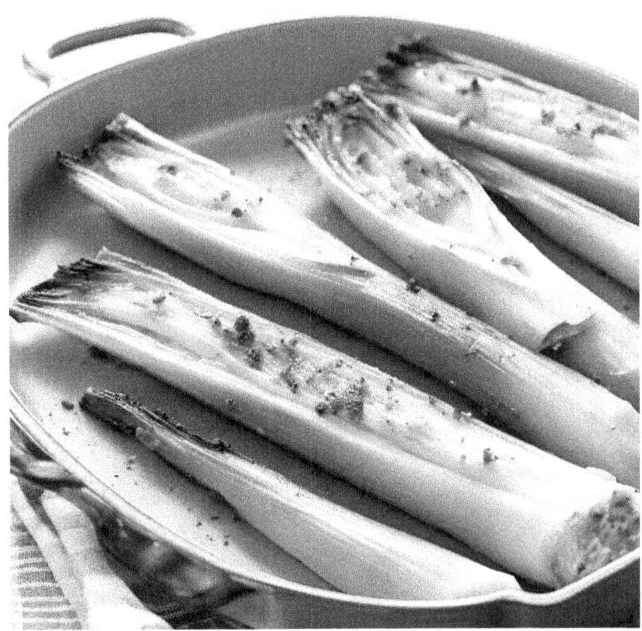

16. Fennel and Apple Salad

Ingredients

- 1 large fennel bulb, thinly sliced
- 2 medium apples, thinly sliced
- 1/4 cup fresh parsley, chopped
- 2 tablespoons olive oil
- 1 tablespoon lemon juice
- 1/4 teaspoon ground black pepper

Instructions

1. In a large bowl, combine the thinly sliced fennel, apples, and chopped parsley.
2. In a small bowl, whisk together the olive oil, lemon juice, and ground black pepper.
3. Pour the dressing over the fennel and apple mixture and toss to coat evenly.
4. Serve immediately.

Nutrition Information (Per Serving)

- Calories: 110
- Protein: 1g
- Carbohydrates: 12g
- Dietary Fiber: 4g
- Sugars: 8g
- Fat: 7g
- Saturated Fat: 1g
- Cholesterol: 0mg
- Sodium: 15mg

Servings

- **4 servings**

Cooking Time

- **10 minutes**

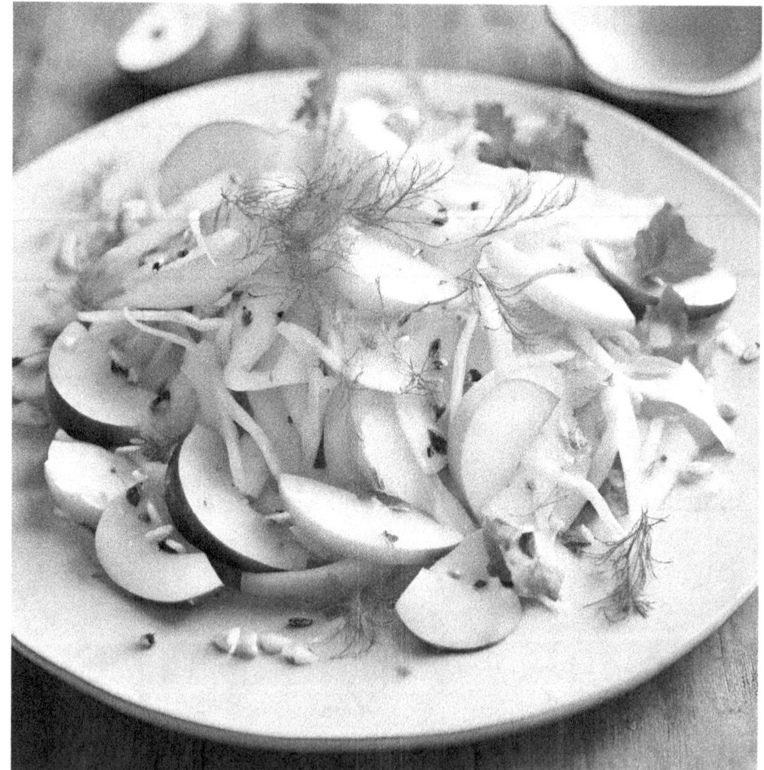

17. Eggplant Caponata

Ingredients

- 1 large eggplant, diced
- 2 celery stalks, diced
- 1/2 cup pitted green olives, chopped
- 1/4 cup capers, rinsed
- 1/4 cup olive oil
- 1/4 cup raisins
- 1 teaspoon dried oregano
- 1/4 teaspoon ground black pepper
- Fresh parsley for garnish (optional)

Instructions

1. In a large skillet, heat the olive oil over medium heat.
2. Add the diced eggplant and celery, and cook for 10-12 minutes, stirring occasionally, until the vegetables are tender.
3. Stir in the chopped olives, capers, raisins, dried oregano, and ground black pepper. Cook for an additional 5 minutes.
4. Remove from heat and let the caponata cool to room temperature.
5. Garnish with fresh parsley if desired and serve.

Nutrition Information (Per Serving)

- Calories: 160
- Protein: 2g
- Carbohydrates: 15g
- Dietary Fiber: 6g
- Sugars: 8g
- Fat: 11g
- Saturated Fat: 1.5g
- Cholesterol: 0mg
- Sodium: 250mg

Servings

- **4 servings**

Cooking Time

- **20 minutes**

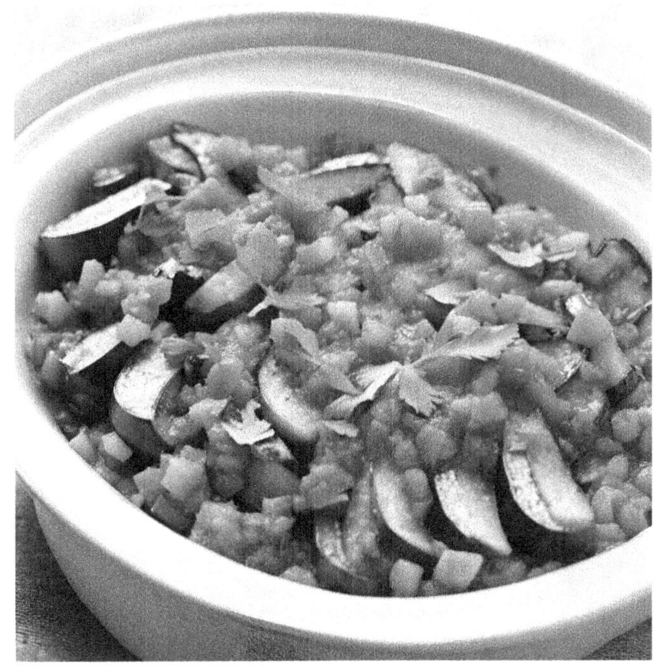

18. Butternut Squash Risotto

Ingredients

- 1 cup Arborio rice
- 2 cups butternut squash, peeled and diced
- 4 cups low-sodium vegetable broth
- 1/2 cup unsweetened almond milk
- 2 tablespoons olive oil
- 1/4 cup grated Parmesan cheese (optional)
- 1 teaspoon dried thyme
- 1/4 teaspoon ground black pepper

Instructions

1. In a medium saucepan, bring the vegetable broth to a simmer and keep warm.
2. In a large skillet, heat the olive oil over medium heat.
3. Add the diced butternut squash and cook for 5-7 minutes, until slightly tender.
4. Stir in the Arborio rice and cook for 2-3 minutes, until lightly toasted.
5. Add 1/2 cup of the warm vegetable broth to the skillet and stir until absorbed. Continue adding the broth 1/2 cup at a time, stirring constantly, until the rice is creamy and cooked through (about 20-25 minutes).
6. Stir in the almond milk, dried thyme, ground black pepper, and Parmesan cheese (if using).
7. Serve immediately.

Nutrition Information (Per Serving)

- Calories: 250
- Protein: 6g
- Carbohydrates: 45g
- Dietary Fiber: 4g
- Sugars: 5g
- Fat: 8g
- Saturated Fat: 1.5g
- Cholesterol: 5mg
- Sodium: 200mg

Servings

- **4 servings**

Cooking Time

- **30 minutes**

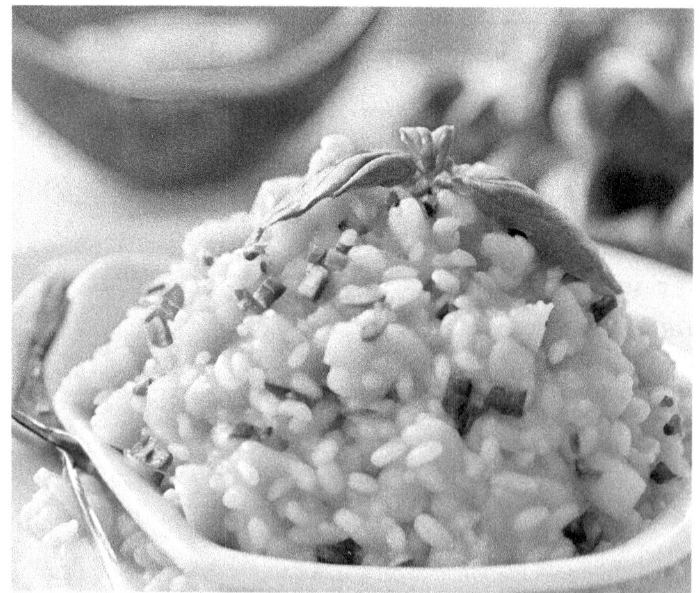

19. Stir-Fried Bok Choy

Ingredients

- 4 cups bok choy, chopped
- 1 tablespoon olive oil
- 1/4 cup low-sodium vegetable broth
- 1 tablespoon soy sauce (low-sodium)
- 1/4 teaspoon ground ginger

Instructions

1. In a large skillet, heat the olive oil over medium heat.
2. Add the chopped bok choy and stir-fry for 2-3 minutes, until it starts to wilt.
3. Add the vegetable broth, soy sauce, and ground ginger.
4. Cook for an additional 3-5 minutes, until the bok choy is tender and the liquid has reduced slightly.
5. Serve immediately.

Nutrition Information (Per Serving)

- Calories: 60
- Protein: 2g
- Carbohydrates: 7g
- Dietary Fiber: 3g
- Sugars: 2g
- Fat: 3g
- Saturated Fat: 0.5g
- Cholesterol: 0mg
- Sodium: 220mg

Servings

- **4 servings**

Cooking Time

- **10 minutes**

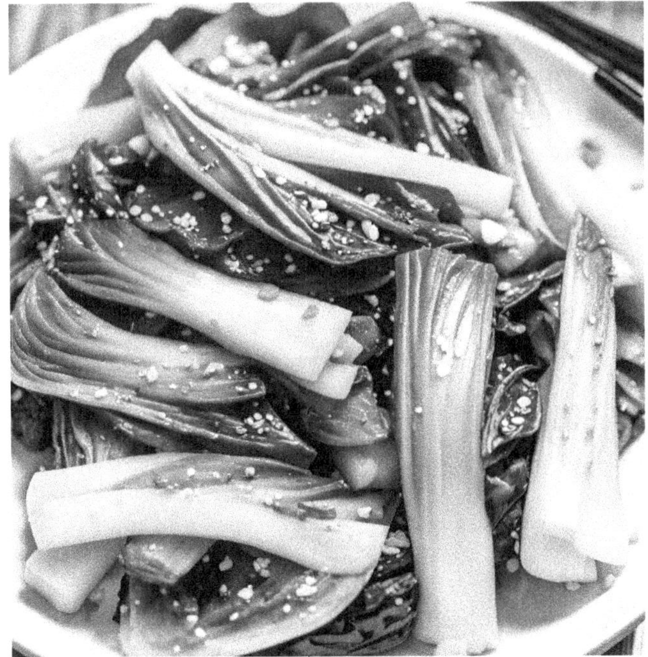

20. Roasted Turnips with Rosemary

Ingredients

- 4 medium turnips, peeled and diced
- 2 tablespoons olive oil
- 1 teaspoon dried rosemary
- 1/4 teaspoon ground black pepper

Instructions

1. Preheat the oven to 400°F (200°C) and line a baking sheet with parchment paper.
2. In a large bowl, toss the diced turnips with olive oil, dried rosemary, and ground black pepper.
3. Spread the turnips evenly on the prepared baking sheet.
4. Roast for 25-30 minutes, or until the turnips are tender and golden brown, stirring halfway through.
5. Serve warm.

Nutrition Information (Per Serving)

- Calories: 90
- Protein: 1g
- Carbohydrates: 11g
- Dietary Fiber: 3g
- Sugars: 5g
- Fat: 5g
- Saturated Fat: 1g
- Cholesterol: 0mg
- Sodium: 15mg

Servings

- **4 servings**

Cooking Time

- **35 minutes**

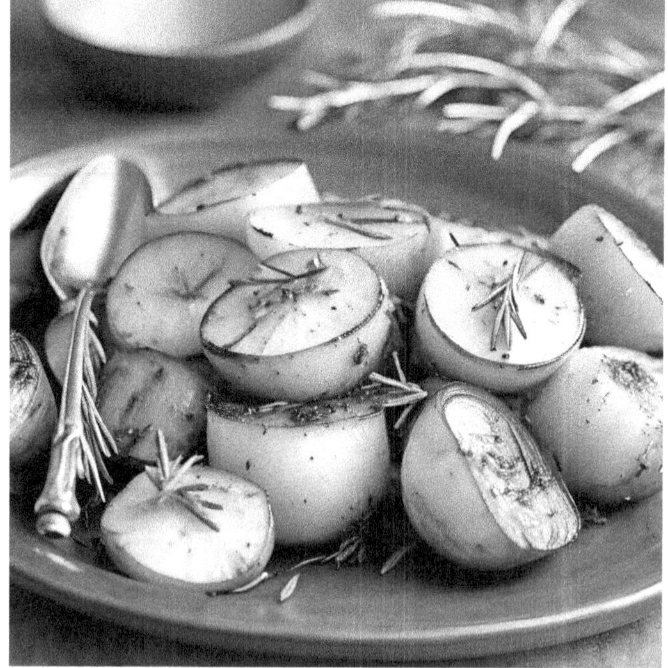

21. Steamed Artichokes

Ingredients

- 4 large artichokes
- 2 tablespoons olive oil
- 1 tablespoon lemon juice
- 1/4 teaspoon ground black pepper

Instructions

1. Trim the stems and tops of the artichokes. Remove the small, tough leaves near the base.
2. Bring a large pot of water to a boil and place a steamer basket over it.
3. Place the artichokes in the steamer basket, cover, and steam for 25-30 minutes, or until the leaves pull away easily.
4. In a small bowl, whisk together the olive oil, lemon juice, and ground black pepper.
5. Drizzle the dressing over the steamed artichokes before serving.

Nutrition Information (Per Serving)

- Calories: 120
- Protein: 4g
- Carbohydrates: 13g
- Dietary Fiber: 7g
- Sugars: 1g
- Fat: 7g
- Saturated Fat: 1g
- Cholesterol: 0mg
- Sodium: 60mg

Servings

- **4 servings**

Cooking Time

- **35 minutes**

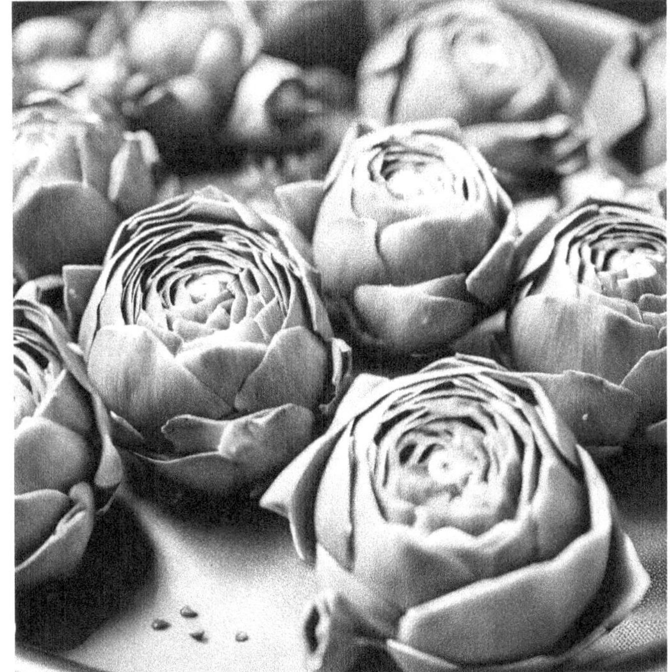

22. Kale Chips

Ingredients

- 1 large bunch of kale, stems removed and leaves torn into bite-sized pieces
- 2 tablespoons olive oil
- 1/4 teaspoon ground black pepper

Instructions

1. Preheat the oven to 300°F (150°C) and line a baking sheet with parchment paper.
2. In a large bowl, toss the kale pieces with olive oil and ground black pepper.
3. Spread the kale evenly on the prepared baking sheet.
4. Bake for 20-25 minutes, or until the kale is crispy, stirring halfway through.
5. Serve immediately.

Nutrition Information (Per Serving)

- Calories: 80
- Protein: 2g
- Carbohydrates: 7g
- Dietary Fiber: 2g
- Sugars: 0g
- Fat: 5g
- Saturated Fat: 1g
- Cholesterol: 0mg
- Sodium: 15mg

Servings

- **4 servings**

Cooking Time

- **30 minutes**

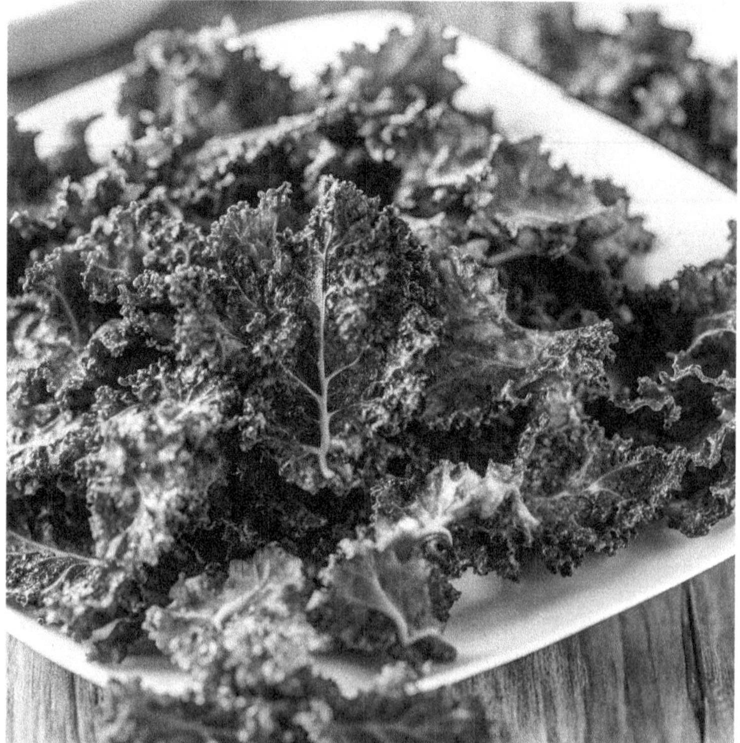

23. Grilled Zucchini and Squash

Ingredients

- 2 medium zucchinis, sliced lengthwise
- 2 medium yellow squashes, sliced lengthwise
- 2 tablespoons olive oil
- 1 tablespoon lemon juice
- 1/4 teaspoon ground black pepper

Instructions

1. Preheat the grill to medium-high heat.
2. In a small bowl, whisk together the olive oil, lemon juice, and ground black pepper.
3. Brush the zucchini and squash slices with the olive oil mixture.
4. Grill the vegetables for 3-4 minutes on each side, until tender and slightly charred.
5. Serve immediately.

Nutrition Information (Per Serving)

- Calories: 70
- Protein: 2g
- Carbohydrates: 6g
- Dietary Fiber: 2g
- Sugars: 4g
- Fat: 5g
- Saturated Fat: 1g
- Cholesterol: 0mg
- Sodium: 10mg

Servings

- **4 servings**

Cooking Time

- **10 minutes**

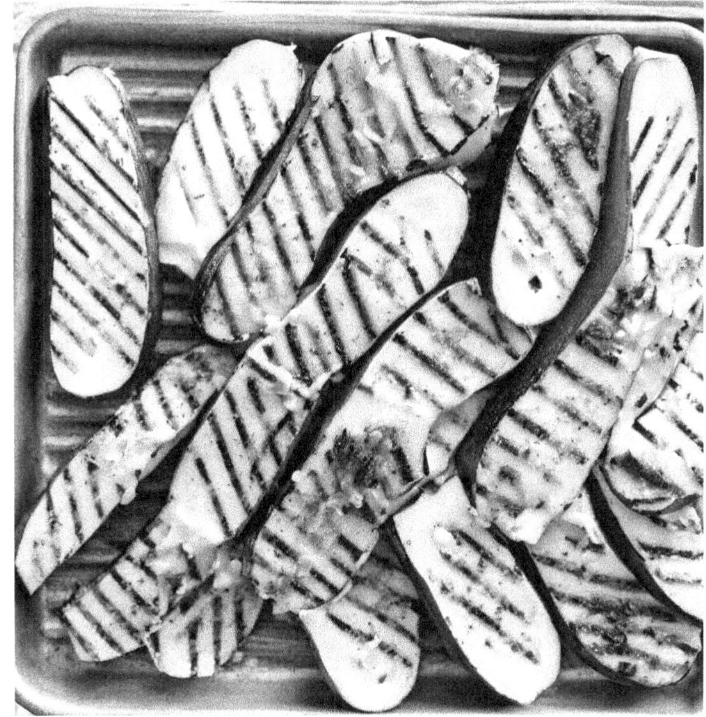

24. Vegetable Quiche

Ingredients

- 1 pre-made whole wheat pie crust
- 1 cup diced mushrooms
- 1 cup chopped spinach
- 1 cup shredded mozzarella cheese
- 4 large eggs
- 1 cup unsweetened almond milk
- 1/2 teaspoon ground black pepper
- 1/2 teaspoon dried thyme

Instructions

1. Preheat the oven to 375°F (190°C).
2. Place the pie crust in a 9-inch pie dish and set aside.
3. In a large bowl, whisk together the eggs, almond milk, ground black pepper, and dried thyme.
4. Layer the diced mushrooms, chopped spinach, and shredded mozzarella cheese in the pie crust.
5. Pour the egg mixture over the vegetables and cheese.
6. Bake for 35-40 minutes, or until the quiche is set and golden brown.
7. Let the quiche cool for 10 minutes before slicing and serving.

Nutrition Information (Per Serving)

- Calories: 220
- Protein: 10g
- Carbohydrates: 18g
- Dietary Fiber: 2g
- Sugars: 1g
- Fat: 13g
- Saturated Fat: 4g
- Cholesterol: 110mg
- Sodium: 250mg

Servings

- **6 servings**

Cooking Time

- **50 minutes**

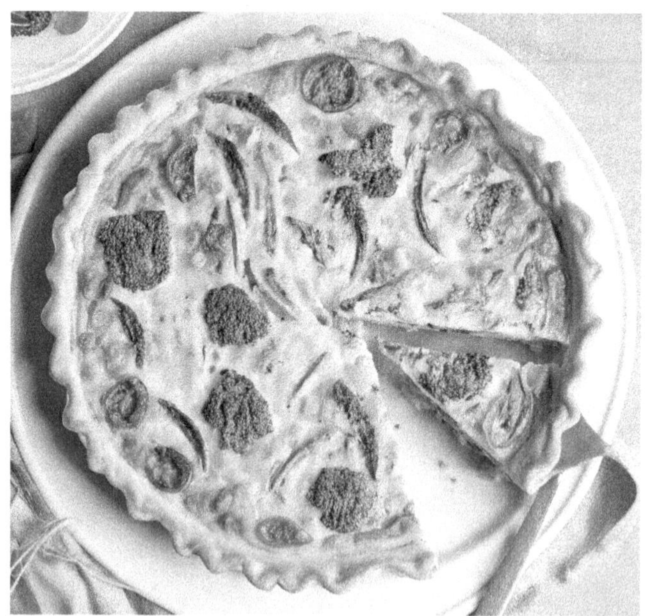

25. Chilled Beet Soup

Ingredients

- 4 medium beets, peeled and diced
- 2 cups low-sodium vegetable broth
- 1 cup unsweetened almond milk
- 2 tablespoons lemon juice
- 1 teaspoon dried dill
- 1/4 teaspoon ground black pepper
- Fresh dill for garnish (optional)

Instructions

1. In a large pot, combine the diced beets and vegetable broth. Bring to a boil, then reduce the heat and simmer for 20-25 minutes, or until the beets are tender.
2. Remove from heat and let cool slightly.
3. Transfer the beets and broth to a blender and add the almond milk, lemon juice, dried dill, and ground black pepper. Blend until smooth.
4. Chill the soup in the refrigerator for at least 2 hours before serving.
5. Garnish with fresh dill if desired.

Nutrition Information (Per Serving)

- Calories: 110
- Protein: 2g
- Carbohydrates: 18g
- Dietary Fiber: 4g
- Sugars: 10g
- Fat: 4g
- Saturated Fat: 0.5g
- Cholesterol: 0mg
- Sodium: 130mg

Servings

- **4 servings**

Cooking Time

- **30 minutes prep, 2 hours chilling**

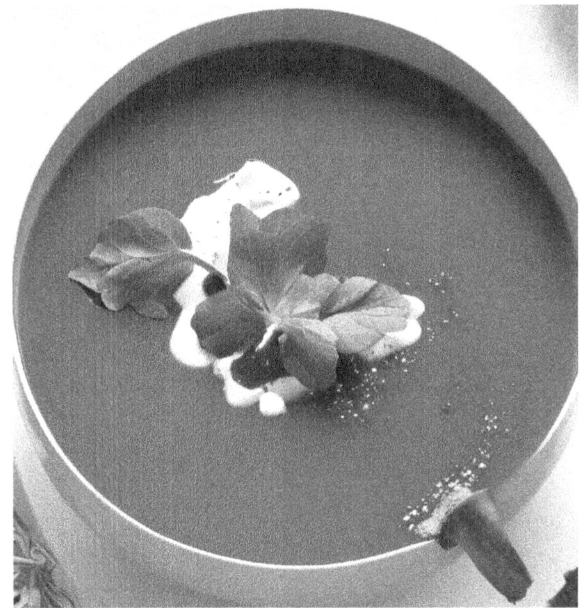

Poultry Recipes

1. Turkey Vegetable Loaf
Ingredients
- 1 pound ground turkey
- 1 cup grated carrots
- 1 cup grated zucchini
- 1/2 cup rolled oats
- 2 large eggs, beaten
- 1/4 cup plain Greek yogurt
- 1 tablespoon dried thyme
- 1/2 teaspoon ground black pepper

Instructions
1. Preheat the oven to 375°F (190°C) and line a loaf pan with parchment paper.
2. In a large bowl, combine the ground turkey, grated carrots, grated zucchini, rolled oats, beaten eggs, Greek yogurt, dried thyme, and ground black pepper. Mix well.
3. Transfer the mixture to the prepared loaf pan and press it down evenly.
4. Bake for 45-50 minutes, or until the internal temperature reaches 165°F (75°C).
5. Let the loaf rest for 10 minutes before slicing and serving.

Nutrition Information (Per Serving)
- Calories: 220
- Protein: 25g
- Carbohydrates: 10g
- Dietary Fiber: 2g
- Sugars: 3g
- Fat: 10g
- Saturated Fat: 2g
- Cholesterol: 110mg
- Sodium: 120mg

Servings
- **6 servings**

Cooking Time
- **60 minutes**

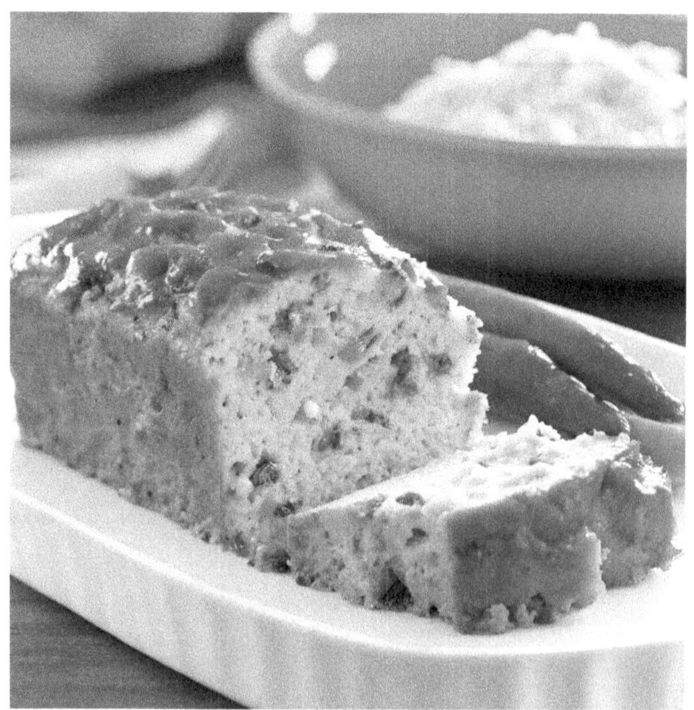

2. Chicken Sweet Potato Hash

Ingredients

- 1 pound boneless, skinless chicken breasts, diced
- 2 large sweet potatoes, peeled and diced
- 1 cup diced celery
- 2 tablespoons olive oil
- 1 teaspoon dried rosemary
- 1/2 teaspoon ground black pepper

Instructions

1. In a large skillet, heat the olive oil over medium heat.
2. Add the diced chicken and cook for 5-7 minutes, until browned and cooked through. Remove the chicken from the skillet and set aside.
3. In the same skillet, add the diced sweet potatoes and celery. Cook for 10-12 minutes, stirring occasionally, until the sweet potatoes are tender.
4. Return the chicken to the skillet and add the dried rosemary and ground black pepper. Stir to combine and cook for an additional 2-3 minutes.
5. Serve immediately.

Nutrition Information (Per Serving)

- Calories: 300
- Protein: 30g
- Carbohydrates: 25g
- Dietary Fiber: 5g
- Sugars: 8g
- Fat: 10g
- Saturated Fat: 1.5g
- Cholesterol: 75mg
- Sodium: 90mg

Servings

- **4 servings**

Cooking Time

- **25 minutes**

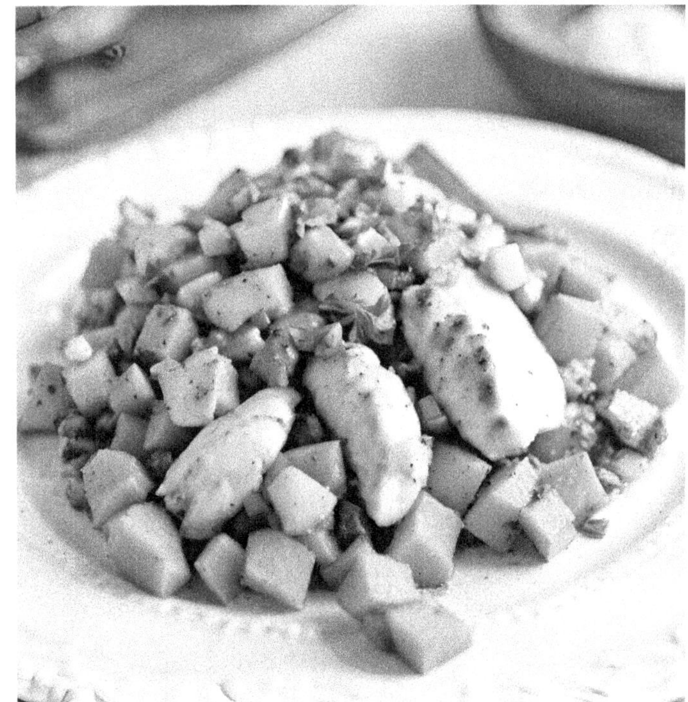

3. Turkey Cranberry Wraps

Ingredients

- 1 pound cooked turkey breast, sliced
- 4 large whole wheat tortillas
- 1/2 cup cranberry sauce (no added sugar)
- 1 cup baby spinach leaves
- 1/4 cup plain Greek yogurt
- 1 tablespoon lemon juice
- 1/4 teaspoon ground black pepper

Instructions

1. In a small bowl, mix the Greek yogurt, lemon juice, and ground black pepper.
2. Lay out the tortillas and spread a thin layer of the yogurt mixture on each one.
3. Top each tortilla with slices of turkey breast, cranberry sauce, and baby spinach leaves.
4. Roll up the tortillas tightly and slice in half before serving.

Nutrition Information (Per Serving)

- Calories: 350
- Protein: 30g
- Carbohydrates: 35g
- Dietary Fiber: 5g
- Sugars: 10g
- Fat: 10g
- Saturated Fat: 2g
- Cholesterol: 70mg
- Sodium: 320mg

Servings

- **4 servings**

Cooking Time

- **10 minutes**

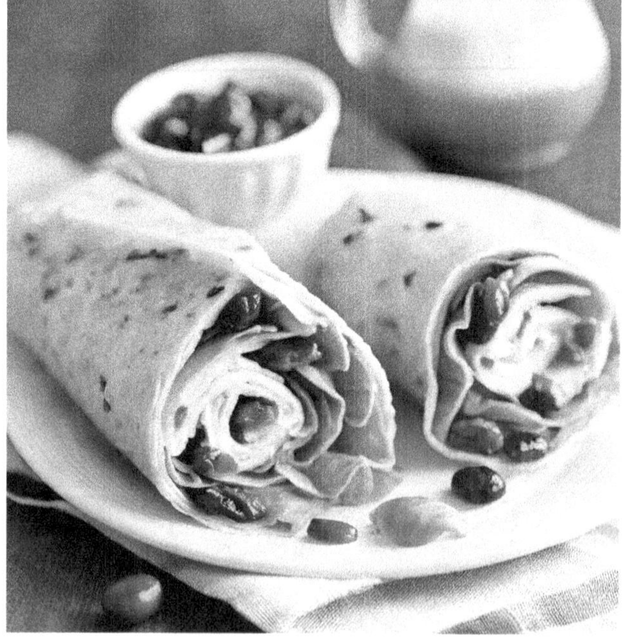

4. Chicken and Barley Stew

Ingredients

- 1 pound boneless, skinless chicken thighs, diced
- 1 cup barley
- 4 cups low-sodium chicken broth
- 2 large carrots, diced
- 2 celery stalks, diced
- 1 cup diced potatoes
- 2 tablespoons olive oil
- 1 teaspoon dried thyme
- 1/2 teaspoon ground black pepper

Instructions

1. In a large pot, heat the olive oil over medium heat.
2. Add the diced chicken thighs and cook for 5-7 minutes, until browned and cooked through. Remove the chicken from the pot and set aside.
3. In the same pot, add the diced carrots, celery, and potatoes. Cook for 5-7 minutes, stirring occasionally.
4. Add the barley, chicken broth, dried thyme, and ground black pepper. Stir to combine and bring to a boil.
5. Reduce the heat to low, cover, and simmer for 30-35 minutes, or until the barley is tender.
6. Return the chicken to the pot and cook for an additional 5 minutes, until heated through.
7. Serve hot.

Nutrition Information (Per Serving)

- Calories: 320
- Protein: 25g
- Carbohydrates: 35g
- Dietary Fiber: 7g
- Sugars: 6g
- Fat: 10g
- Saturated Fat: 2g
- Cholesterol: 75mg
- Sodium: 200mg

Servings

- **4 servings**

Cooking Time

- **45 minutes**

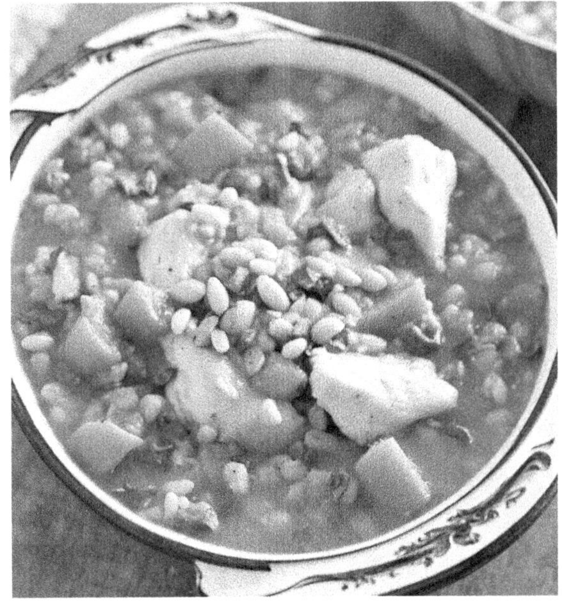

5. Turkey in Creamy Mushroom Sauce

Ingredients

- 1 pound turkey breast, thinly sliced
- 2 cups sliced mushrooms
- 1 cup low-sodium chicken broth
- 1/2 cup unsweetened almond milk
- 2 tablespoons olive oil
- 1 tablespoon cornstarch mixed with 2 tablespoons water
- 1 teaspoon dried thyme
- 1/4 teaspoon ground black pepper

Instructions

1. In a large skillet, heat the olive oil over medium heat.
2. Add the turkey slices and cook for 3-4 minutes on each side, until golden brown and cooked through. Remove the turkey from the skillet and set aside.
3. In the same skillet, add the sliced mushrooms and cook for 5-7 minutes, until they release their juices and begin to brown.
4. Add the chicken broth and dried thyme to the skillet. Bring to a simmer.
5. Stir in the almond milk and the cornstarch mixture. Cook for 2-3 minutes, stirring constantly, until the sauce thickens.
6. Return the turkey to the skillet and cook for an additional 2-3 minutes, until heated through.
7. Sprinkle with ground black pepper before serving.

Nutrition Information (Per Serving)

- Calories: 250
- Protein: 28g
- Carbohydrates: 6g
- Dietary Fiber: 1g
- Sugars: 2g
- Fat: 12g
- Saturated Fat: 2g
- Cholesterol: 65mg
- Sodium: 160mg

Servings

- **4 servings**

Cooking Time

- **20 minutes**

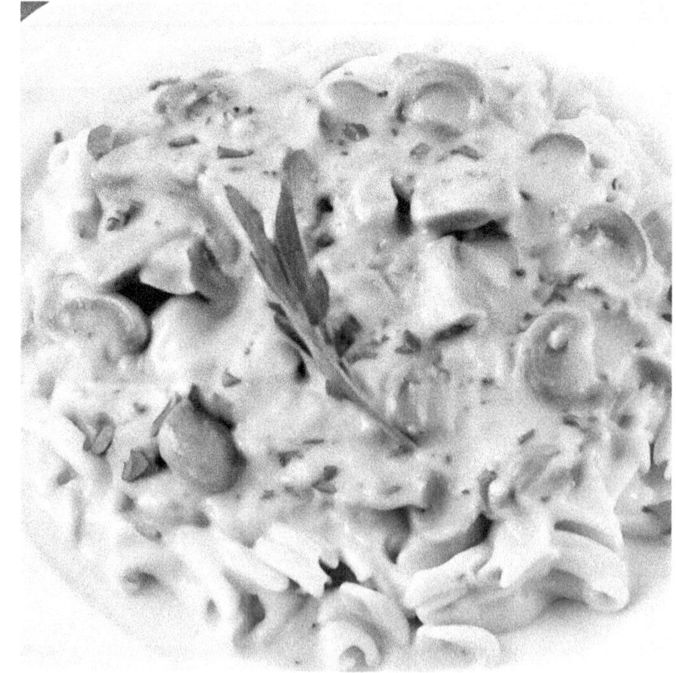

6. Grilled Chicken with Avocado Salad

Ingredients

- 1 pound boneless, skinless chicken breasts
- 2 tablespoons olive oil
- 1 tablespoon lemon juice
- 1 teaspoon dried oregano
- 1/4 teaspoon ground black pepper
- 2 avocados, diced
- 1 cup cherry tomatoes, halved
- 1/4 cup chopped fresh cilantro
- 1 tablespoon lime juice

Instructions

1. Preheat the grill to medium-high heat.
2. In a small bowl, mix the olive oil, lemon juice, dried oregano, and ground black pepper. Brush the mixture over the chicken breasts.
3. Grill the chicken for 5-7 minutes on each side, until the internal temperature reaches 165°F (75°C). Remove from the grill and let rest for 5 minutes before slicing.
4. In a large bowl, combine the diced avocados, cherry tomatoes, and chopped cilantro.
5. Drizzle with lime juice and toss gently to combine.
6. Serve the grilled chicken slices with the avocado salad.

Nutrition Information (Per Serving)

- Calories: 320
- Protein: 30g
- Carbohydrates: 12g
- Dietary Fiber: 7g
- Sugars: 2g
- Fat: 18g
- Saturated Fat: 3g
- Cholesterol: 70mg
- Sodium: 200mg

Servings

- **4 servings**

Cooking Time

- **20 minutes**

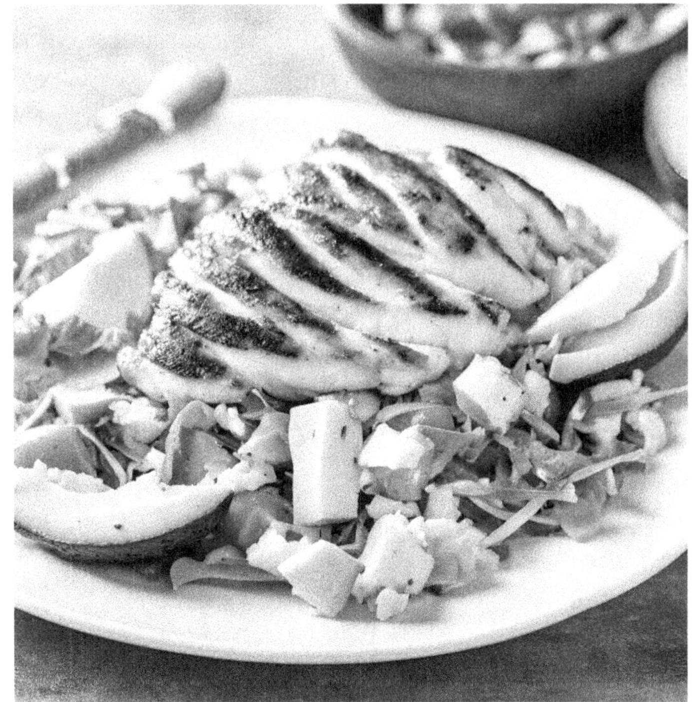

7. Chicken Minestrone Soup

Ingredients

- 1 pound boneless, skinless chicken thighs, diced
- 1 cup diced carrots
- 1 cup diced zucchini
- 1 cup diced celery
- 1 cup canned kidney beans, rinsed and drained
- 1/2 cup uncooked pasta (small shapes)
- 4 cups low-sodium chicken broth
- 2 tablespoons olive oil
- 1 teaspoon dried basil
- 1/4 teaspoon ground black pepper
- 1/4 cup grated Parmesan cheese (optional)

Instructions

1. In a large pot, heat the olive oil over medium heat.
2. Add the diced chicken thighs and cook for 5-7 minutes, until browned and cooked through. Remove the chicken from the pot and set aside.
3. In the same pot, add the diced carrots, zucchini, and celery. Cook for 5-7 minutes, stirring occasionally.
4. Add the chicken broth, kidney beans, and pasta. Bring to a boil, then reduce the heat and simmer for 10-12 minutes, or until the pasta is cooked and the vegetables are tender.
5. Return the chicken to the pot and stir in the dried basil and ground black pepper. Cook for an additional 5 minutes.
6. Serve hot, sprinkled with grated Parmesan cheese if desired.

Nutrition Information (Per Serving)

- Calories: 290
- Protein: 25g
- Carbohydrates: 25g
- Dietary Fiber: 5g
- Sugars: 4g
- Fat: 10g
- Saturated Fat: 2g
- Cholesterol: 70mg
- Sodium: 240mg

Servings

- **4 servings**

Cooking Time

- **40 minutes**

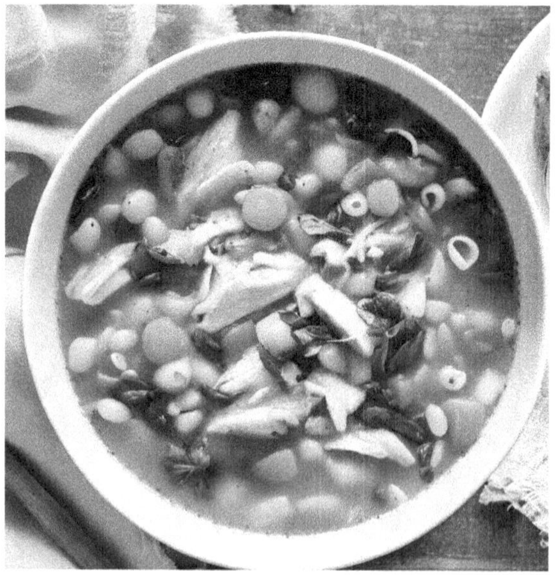

8. Stuffed Chicken Breasts

Ingredients

- 4 boneless, skinless chicken breasts
- 1 cup fresh spinach, chopped
- 1/2 cup ricotta cheese
- 1/4 cup grated Parmesan cheese
- 1 teaspoon dried oregano
- 1/2 teaspoon ground black pepper
- 2 tablespoons olive oil

Instructions

1. Preheat the oven to 375°F (190°C) and line a baking sheet with parchment paper.
2. In a bowl, mix the chopped spinach, ricotta cheese, Parmesan cheese, dried oregano, and ground black pepper.
3. Cut a pocket into the side of each chicken breast and stuff with the spinach mixture.
4. Secure with toothpicks if necessary.
5. Heat the olive oil in a large skillet over medium heat.
6. Sear the stuffed chicken breasts for 3-4 minutes on each side, until golden brown.
7. Transfer the chicken to the prepared baking sheet and bake for 20-25 minutes, until cooked through and the internal temperature reaches 165°F (75°C).
8. Serve warm.

Nutrition Information (Per Serving)

- Calories: 300
- Protein: 35g
- Carbohydrates: 2g
- Dietary Fiber: 1g
- Sugars: 0g
- Fat: 16g
- Saturated Fat: 5g
- Cholesterol: 110mg
- Sodium: 250mg

Servings

- **4 servings**

Cooking Time

- **35 minutes**

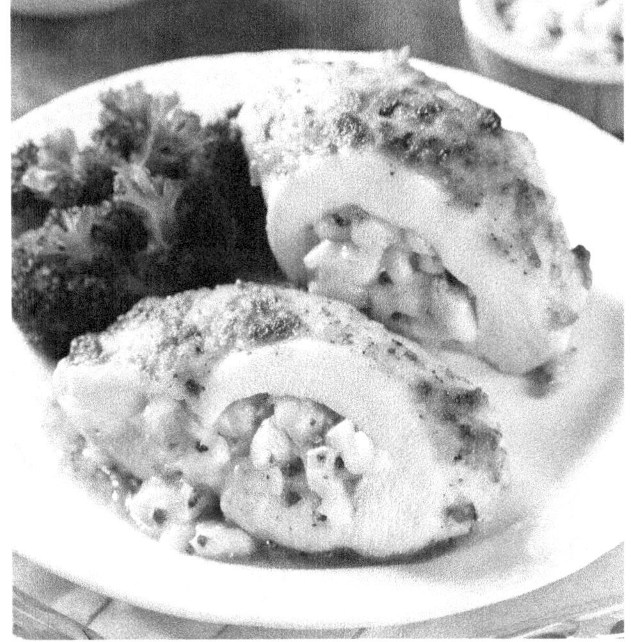

9. Turkey Bolognese

Ingredients

- 1 pound ground turkey
- 1 cup diced carrots
- 1 cup diced celery
- 2 cups low-sodium vegetable broth
- 1 cup unsweetened almond milk
- 1 teaspoon dried basil
- 1 teaspoon dried oregano
- 1/4 teaspoon ground black pepper
- 2 tablespoons olive oil
- Whole wheat pasta, cooked according to package instructions

Instructions

1. In a large skillet, heat the olive oil over medium heat.
2. Add the ground turkey and cook for 5-7 minutes, until browned and cooked through.
3. Add the diced carrots and celery, and cook for 5 minutes, until slightly tender.
4. Stir in the vegetable broth, almond milk, dried basil, dried oregano, and ground black pepper.
5. Bring to a simmer and cook for 20-25 minutes, until the sauce thickens.
6. Serve the turkey bolognese over whole wheat pasta.

Nutrition Information (Per Serving)

- Calories: 350
- Protein: 30g
- Carbohydrates: 25g
- Dietary Fiber: 4g
- Sugars: 6g
- Fat: 15g
- Saturated Fat: 3g
- Cholesterol: 80mg
- Sodium: 280mg

Servings

- **4 servings**

Cooking Time

- **35 minutes**

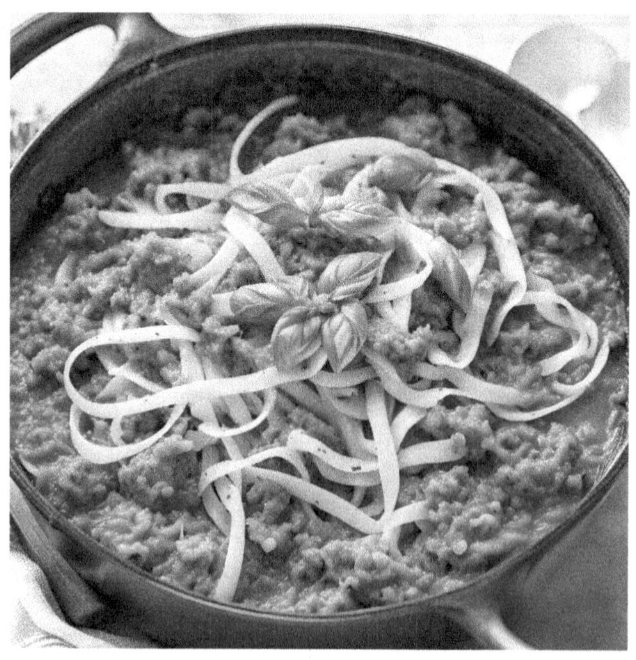

10. Roasted Chicken with Root Vegetables

Ingredients

- 1 whole chicken (about 4 pounds)
- 4 large carrots, peeled and chopped
- 4 medium parsnips, peeled and chopped
- 2 large sweet potatoes, peeled and chopped
- 1/4 cup olive oil
- 1 tablespoon dried rosemary
- 1/4 teaspoon ground black pepper

Instructions

1. Preheat the oven to 400°F (200°C) and line a roasting pan with parchment paper.
2. In a large bowl, toss the chopped carrots, parsnips, and sweet potatoes with half of the olive oil, dried rosemary, and ground black pepper.
3. Place the vegetables in the roasting pan.
4. Rub the remaining olive oil over the chicken and season with ground black pepper.
5. Place the chicken on top of the vegetables.
6. Roast for 1 hour and 15 minutes, or until the internal temperature of the chicken reaches 165°F (75°C) and the vegetables are tender.
7. Let the chicken rest for 10 minutes before carving and serving with the roasted vegetables.

Nutrition Information (Per Serving)

- Calories: 450
- Protein: 35g
- Carbohydrates: 30g
- Dietary Fiber: 6g
- Sugars: 10g
- Fat: 20g
- Saturated Fat: 5g
- Cholesterol: 120mg
- Sodium: 140mg

Servings

- **6 servings**

Cooking Time

- **1 hour 30 minutes**

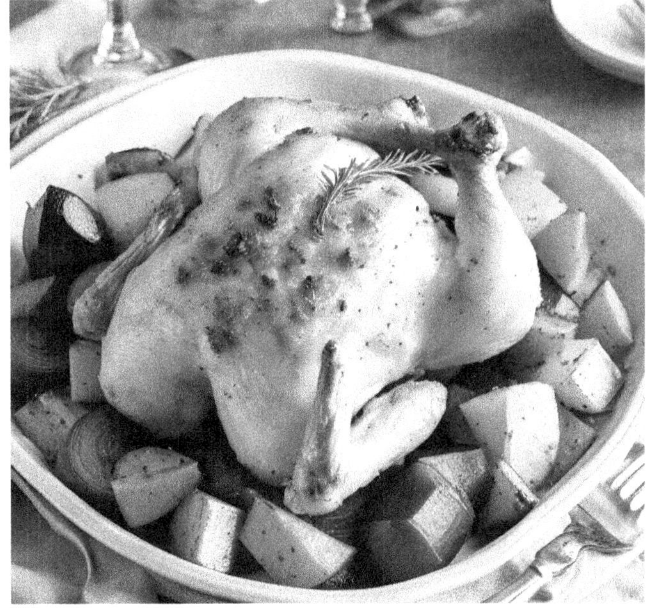

11. Turkey Pot Pie

Ingredients

- 1 pound cooked turkey breast, diced
- 2 cups diced carrots
- 1 cup diced celery
- 1 cup frozen peas
- 1/2 cup unsweetened almond milk
- 1/2 cup low-sodium chicken broth
- 2 tablespoons olive oil
- 1 teaspoon dried thyme
- 1/4 teaspoon ground black pepper
- 1 sheet puff pastry, thawed

Instructions

1. Preheat the oven to 375°F (190°C).
2. In a large skillet, heat the olive oil over medium heat.
3. Add the diced carrots and celery, and cook for 5-7 minutes, until slightly tender.
4. Stir in the almond milk, chicken broth, dried thyme, and ground black pepper.
5. Add the diced turkey and frozen peas, and cook for an additional 5 minutes.
6. Transfer the mixture to a pie dish.
7. Place the puff pastry sheet over the top of the pie dish and trim any excess.
8. Bake for 25-30 minutes, or until the pastry is golden brown and the filling is bubbling.
9. Let the pot pie cool for 10 minutes before serving.

Nutrition Information (Per Serving)

- Calories: 350
- Protein: 25g
- Carbohydrates: 25g
- Dietary Fiber: 4g
- Sugars: 5g
- Fat: 15g
- Saturated Fat: 4g
- Cholesterol: 70mg
- Sodium: 240mg

Servings

- **6 servings**

Cooking Time

- **45 minutes**

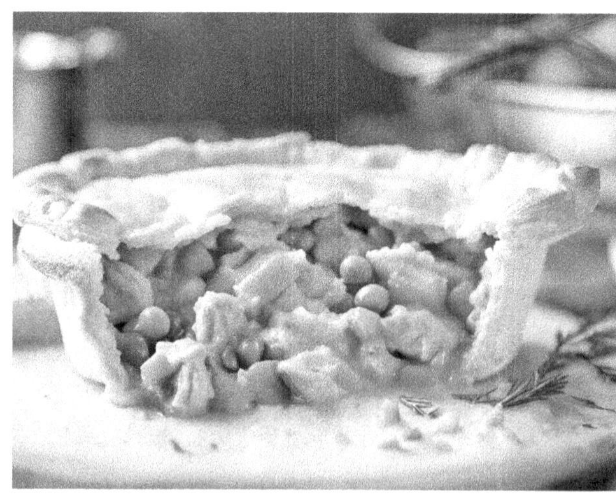

12. Chicken with Mushrooms

Ingredients

- 4 boneless, skinless chicken breasts
- 2 cups sliced mushrooms
- 1 cup low-sodium chicken broth
- 1/2 cup unsweetened almond milk
- 2 tablespoons olive oil
- 1 tablespoon cornstarch mixed with 2 tablespoons water
- 1 teaspoon dried thyme
- 1/4 teaspoon ground black pepper

Instructions

1. In a large skillet, heat the olive oil over medium heat.
2. Add the chicken breasts and cook for 5-7 minutes on each side, until golden brown and cooked through. Remove the chicken from the skillet and set aside.
3. In the same skillet, add the sliced mushrooms and cook for 5-7 minutes, until they release their juices and begin to brown.
4. Add the chicken broth and dried thyme to the skillet. Bring to a simmer.
5. Stir in the almond milk and the cornstarch mixture. Cook for 2-3 minutes, stirring constantly, until the sauce thickens.
6. Return the chicken to the skillet and cook for an additional 2-3 minutes, until heated through.
7. Sprinkle with ground black pepper before serving.

Nutrition Information (Per Serving)

- Calories: 280
- Protein: 35g
- Carbohydrates: 5g
- Dietary Fiber: 1g
- Sugars: 1g
- Fat: 14g
- Saturated Fat: 3g
- Cholesterol: 85mg
- Sodium: 140mg

Servings

- **4 servings**

Cooking Time

- **25 minutes**

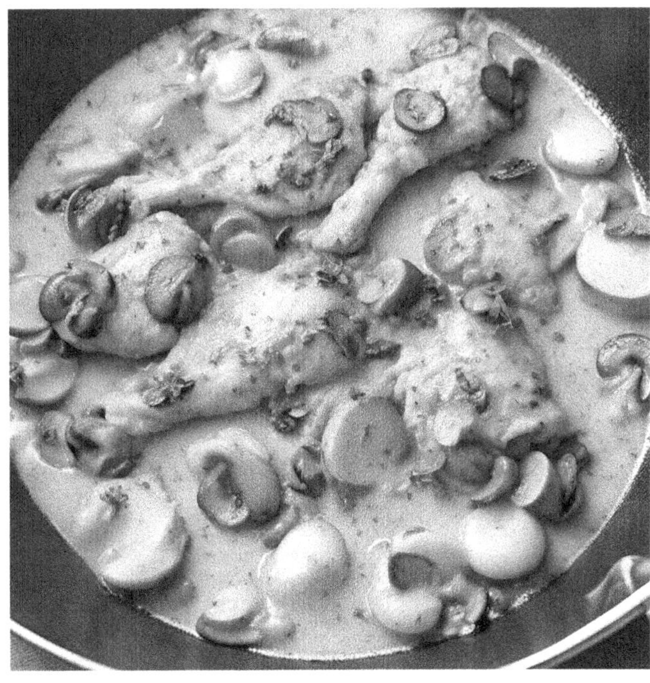

13. Turkey and Apple Stew

Ingredients

- 1 pound turkey breast, cubed
- 2 medium apples, peeled, cored, and diced
- 2 large carrots, diced
- 2 celery stalks, diced
- 4 cups low-sodium chicken broth
- 1/2 cup unsweetened almond milk
- 2 tablespoons olive oil
- 1 teaspoon dried thyme
- 1/2 teaspoon ground black pepper

Instructions

1. In a large pot, heat the olive oil over medium heat.
2. Add the cubed turkey and cook for 5-7 minutes, until browned and cooked through. Remove from the pot and set aside.
3. In the same pot, add the diced carrots and celery. Cook for 5 minutes, stirring occasionally.
4. Add the apples, chicken broth, dried thyme, and ground black pepper. Bring to a boil, then reduce the heat and simmer for 20 minutes, until the vegetables are tender.
5. Stir in the almond milk and return the turkey to the pot. Cook for an additional 5 minutes.
6. Serve hot.

Nutrition Information (Per Serving)

- Calories: 280
- Protein: 30g
- Carbohydrates: 18g
- Dietary Fiber: 4g
- Sugars: 10g
- Fat: 10g
- Saturated Fat: 1.5g
- Cholesterol: 65mg
- Sodium: 160mg

Servings

- **4 servings**

Cooking Time

- **35 minutes**

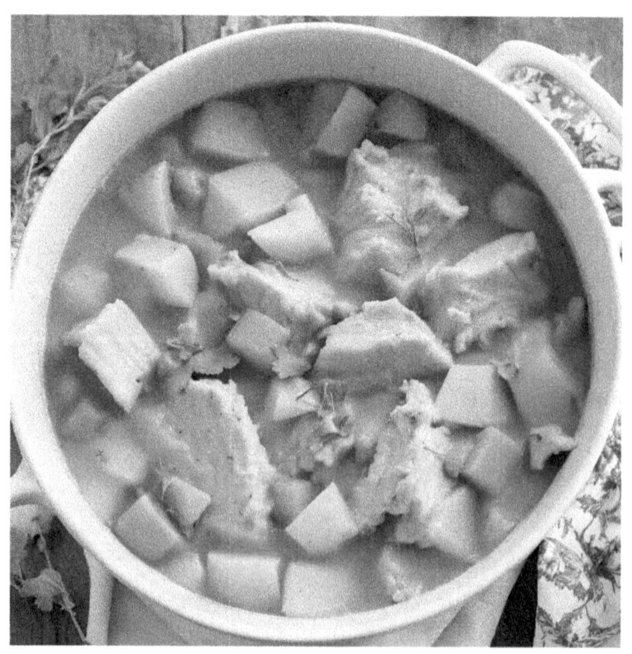

14. Creamy Chicken Alfredo

Ingredients

- 1 pound boneless, skinless chicken breasts, sliced
- 8 ounces whole wheat fettuccine
- 1 cup unsweetened almond milk
- 1/2 cup grated Parmesan cheese
- 1/2 cup plain Greek yogurt
- 2 tablespoons olive oil
- 1 teaspoon dried basil
- 1/4 teaspoon ground black pepper

Instructions

1. Cook the fettuccine according to package instructions. Drain and set aside.
2. In a large skillet, heat the olive oil over medium heat.
3. Add the sliced chicken breasts and cook for 5-7 minutes, until browned and cooked through. Remove from the skillet and set aside.
4. In the same skillet, add the almond milk and bring to a simmer.
5. Stir in the Parmesan cheese, Greek yogurt, dried basil, and ground black pepper. Cook for 2-3 minutes, stirring constantly, until the sauce thickens.
6. Return the chicken to the skillet and cook for an additional 2 minutes.
7. Toss the cooked fettuccine with the sauce and chicken.
8. Serve hot.

Nutrition Information (Per Serving)

- Calories: 400
- Protein: 40g
- Carbohydrates: 30g
- Dietary Fiber: 5g
- Sugars: 3g
- Fat: 15g
- Saturated Fat: 4g
- Cholesterol: 90mg
- Sodium: 260mg

Servings

- **4 servings**

Cooking Time

- **25 minutes**

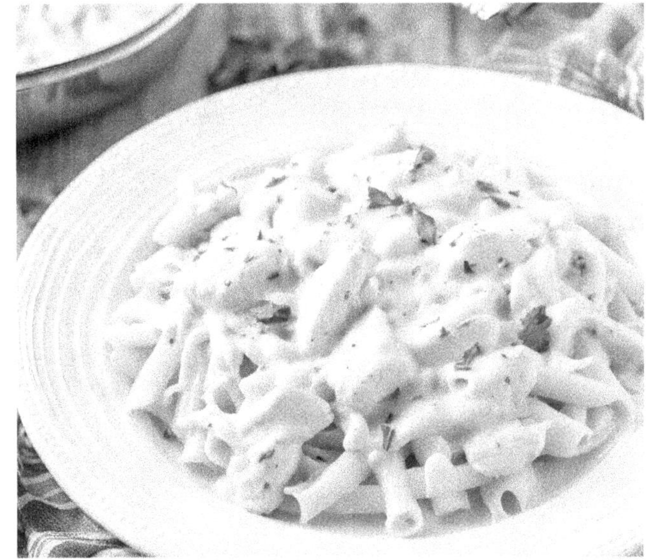

15. Grilled Turkey Tenderloin

Ingredients

- 1 pound turkey tenderloin
- 2 tablespoons olive oil
- 1 tablespoon lemon juice
- 1 teaspoon dried rosemary
- 1/4 teaspoon ground black pepper

Instructions

1. In a small bowl, mix the olive oil, lemon juice, dried rosemary, and ground black pepper.
2. Brush the mixture over the turkey tenderloin.
3. Preheat the grill to medium-high heat.
4. Grill the turkey tenderloin for 5-7 minutes on each side, until the internal temperature reaches 165°F (75°C).
5. Let the turkey rest for 5 minutes before slicing.
6. Serve hot.

Nutrition Information (Per Serving)

- Calories: 200
- Protein: 30g
- Carbohydrates: 0g
- Dietary Fiber: 0g
- Sugars: 0g
- Fat: 8g
- Saturated Fat: 1.5g
- Cholesterol: 70mg
- Sodium: 100mg

Servings

- **4 servings**

Cooking Time

- **20 minutes**

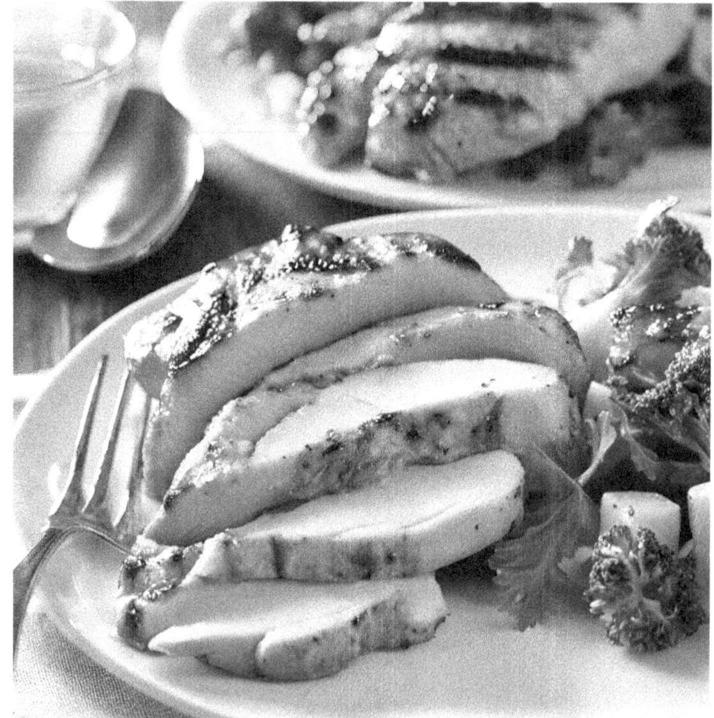

16. Turkey Oatmeal Meatballs

Ingredients

- 1 pound ground turkey
- 1/2 cup rolled oats
- 1/4 cup plain Greek yogurt
- 1 large egg, beaten
- 1 tablespoon dried parsley
- 1 teaspoon dried thyme
- 1/4 teaspoon ground black pepper

Instructions

1. Preheat the oven to 375°F (190°C) and line a baking sheet with parchment paper.
2. In a large bowl, mix the ground turkey, rolled oats, Greek yogurt, beaten egg, dried parsley, dried thyme, and ground black pepper until well combined.
3. Form the mixture into meatballs and place them on the prepared baking sheet.
4. Bake for 20-25 minutes, until the meatballs are cooked through and golden brown.
5. Serve hot.

Nutrition Information (Per Serving)

- Calories: 180
- Protein: 25g
- Carbohydrates: 6g
- Dietary Fiber: 1g
- Sugars: 1g
- Fat: 7g
- Saturated Fat: 1.5g
- Cholesterol: 70mg
- Sodium: 110mg

Servings

- **4 servings**

Cooking Time

- **25 minutes**

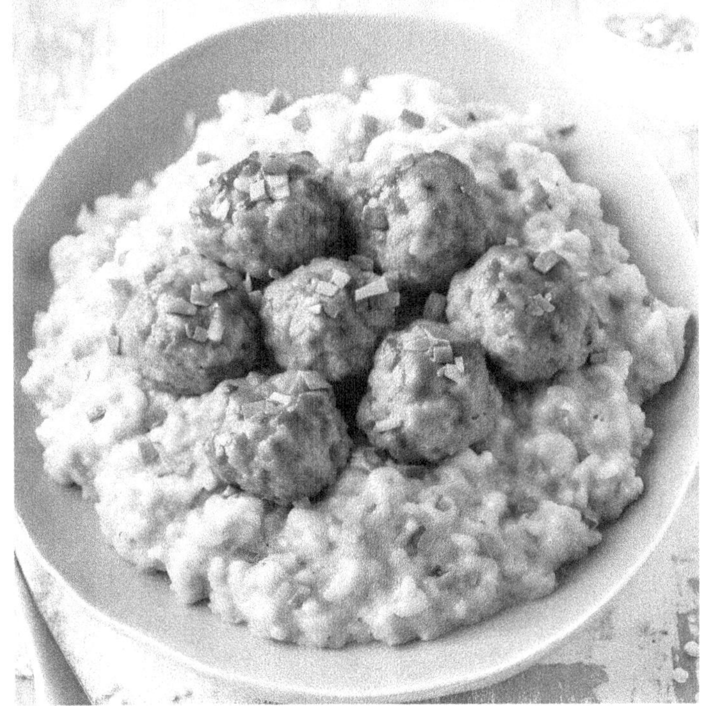

17. Chicken with Parsley Pesto

Ingredients

- 4 boneless, skinless chicken breasts
- 2 cups fresh parsley leaves
- 1/4 cup pine nuts
- 1/4 cup grated Parmesan cheese
- 1/4 cup olive oil
- 1 tablespoon lemon juice
- 1/4 teaspoon ground black pepper

Instructions

1. In a food processor, combine the parsley leaves, pine nuts, Parmesan cheese, olive oil, lemon juice, and ground black pepper. Process until smooth to make the parsley pesto.
2. Preheat the oven to 375°F (190°C) and line a baking sheet with parchment paper.
3. Place the chicken breasts on the prepared baking sheet.
4. Spread the parsley pesto evenly over the chicken breasts.
5. Bake for 20-25 minutes, until the chicken is cooked through and the internal temperature reaches 165°F (75°C).
6. Serve hot.

Nutrition Information (Per Serving)

- Calories: 300
- Protein: 35g
- Carbohydrates: 3g
- Dietary Fiber: 1g
- Sugars: 0g
- Fat: 17g
- Saturated Fat: 3g
- Cholesterol: 85mg
- Sodium: 140mg

Servings

- **4 servings**

Cooking Time

- **30 minutes**

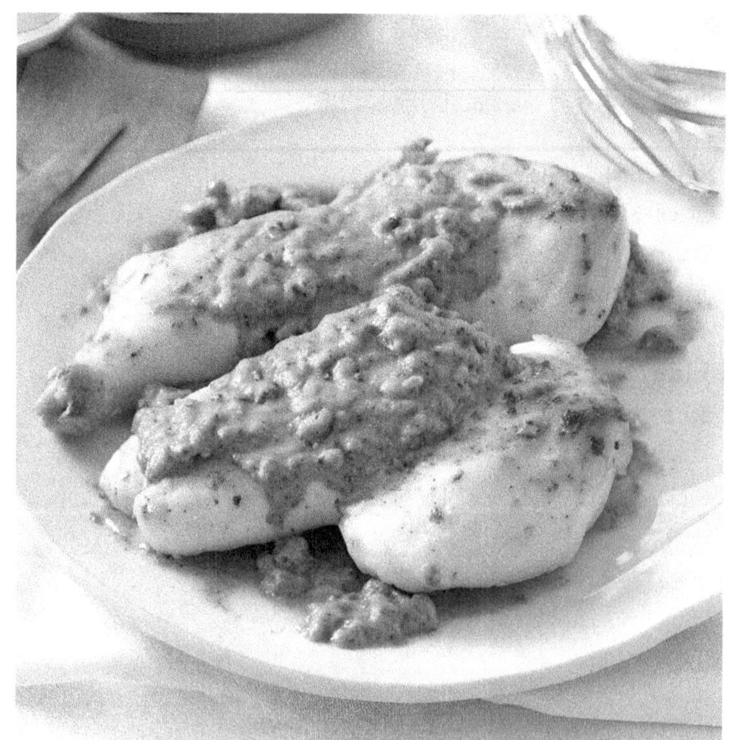

18. Turkey and Carrot Patties

Ingredients

- 1 pound ground turkey
- 1 cup grated carrots
- 1/2 cup rolled oats
- 1 large egg, beaten
- 1/4 cup plain Greek yogurt
- 1 teaspoon dried thyme
- 1/4 teaspoon ground black pepper
- 2 tablespoons olive oil

Instructions

1. In a large bowl, combine the ground turkey, grated carrots, rolled oats, beaten egg, Greek yogurt, dried thyme, and ground black pepper. Mix until well combined.
2. Form the mixture into patties.
3. Heat the olive oil in a large skillet over medium heat.
4. Cook the patties for 4-5 minutes on each side, until golden brown and cooked through.
5. Serve warm.

Nutrition Information (Per Serving)

- Calories: 200
- Protein: 25g
- Carbohydrates: 8g
- Dietary Fiber: 2g
- Sugars: 2g
- Fat: 9g
- Saturated Fat: 2g
- Cholesterol: 75mg
- Sodium: 90mg

Servings

- **4 servings**

Cooking Time

- **20 minutes**

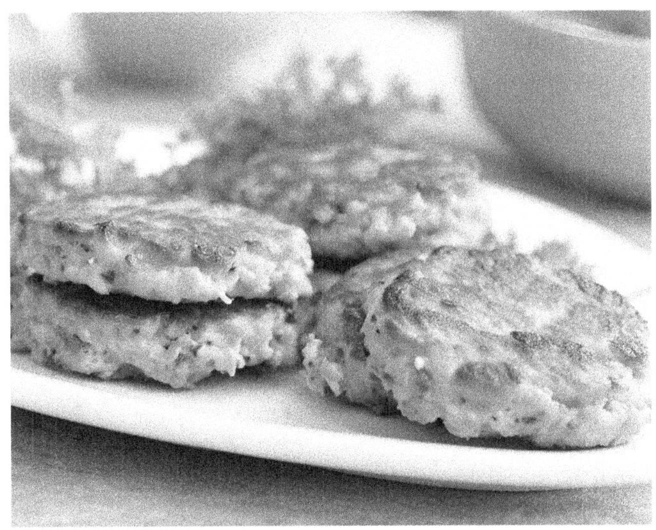

19. Chicken Pilaf

Ingredients

- 1 pound boneless, skinless chicken thighs, diced
- 1 cup brown rice
- 2 cups low-sodium chicken broth
- 1 cup diced carrots
- 1 cup diced celery
- 1/4 cup dried cranberries
- 2 tablespoons olive oil
- 1 teaspoon dried thyme
- 1/4 teaspoon ground black pepper

Instructions

1. In a large pot, heat the olive oil over medium heat.
2. Add the diced chicken thighs and cook for 5-7 minutes, until browned and cooked through. Remove from the pot and set aside.
3. In the same pot, add the brown rice and cook for 2 minutes, stirring frequently.
4. Add the chicken broth, diced carrots, celery, dried cranberries, dried thyme, and ground black pepper. Bring to a boil.
5. Reduce the heat to low, cover, and simmer for 30-35 minutes, or until the rice is tender and the liquid is absorbed.
6. Return the chicken to the pot and stir to combine.
7. Serve warm.

Nutrition Information (Per Serving)

- Calories: 300
- Protein: 25g
- Carbohydrates: 35g
- Dietary Fiber: 4g
- Sugars: 5g
- Fat: 8g
- Saturated Fat: 2g
- Cholesterol: 75mg
- Sodium: 200mg

Servings

- **4 servings**

Cooking Time

- **40 minutes**

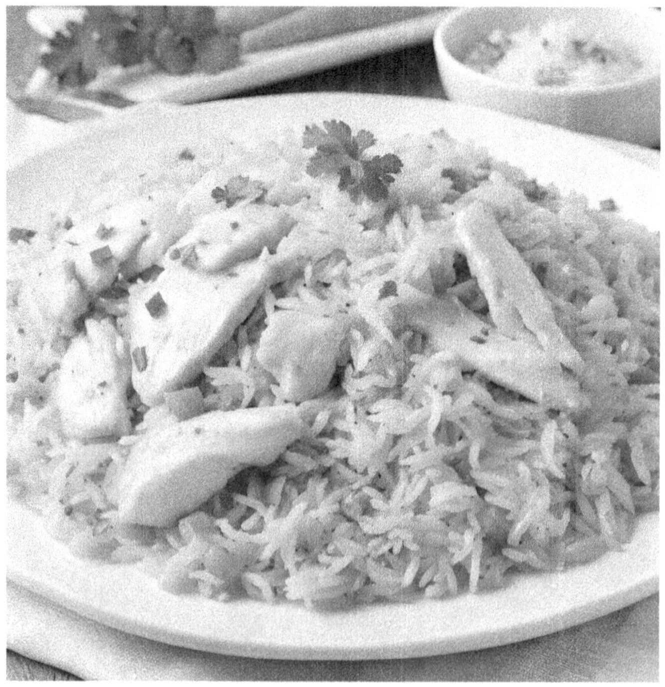

20. Herbed Turkey Steaks

Ingredients

- 4 turkey steaks
- 2 tablespoons olive oil
- 1 tablespoon lemon juice
- 1 teaspoon dried rosemary
- 1 teaspoon dried thyme
- 1/4 teaspoon ground black pepper

Instructions

1. In a small bowl, mix the olive oil, lemon juice, dried rosemary, dried thyme, and ground black pepper.
2. Brush the mixture over the turkey steaks.
3. Preheat a grill or grill pan to medium-high heat.
4. Grill the turkey steaks for 5-6 minutes on each side, until cooked through and the internal temperature reaches 165°F (75°C).
5. Serve warm.

Nutrition Information (Per Serving)

- Calories: 220
- Protein: 30g
- Carbohydrates: 1g
- Dietary Fiber: 0g
- Sugars: 0g
- Fat: 10g
- Saturated Fat: 2g
- Cholesterol: 75mg
- Sodium: 90mg

Servings

- **4 servings**

Cooking Time

- **15 minutes**

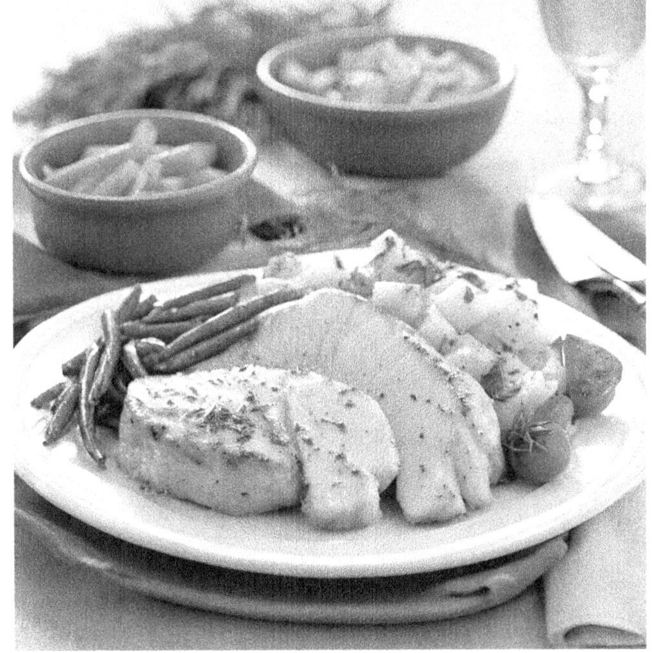

21. Chicken and Rice Porridge

Ingredients

- 1 cup jasmine rice
- 6 cups low-sodium chicken broth
- 1 pound boneless, skinless chicken breasts
- 1 cup diced carrots
- 1 cup diced celery
- 1 teaspoon ground ginger
- 1/4 cup chopped fresh parsley

Instructions

1. In a large pot, combine the jasmine rice and chicken broth. Bring to a boil, then reduce the heat and simmer for 15 minutes.
2. Add the chicken breasts, diced carrots, celery, and ground ginger. Continue to simmer for 25-30 minutes, or until the rice is very soft and the chicken is cooked through.
3. Remove the chicken from the pot, shred it with two forks, and return it to the pot.
4. Stir in the chopped parsley and cook for an additional 5 minutes.
5. Serve warm.

Nutrition Information (Per Serving)

- Calories: 250
- Protein: 28g
- Carbohydrates: 30g
- Dietary Fiber: 2g
- Sugars: 2g
- Fat: 4g
- Saturated Fat: 1g
- Cholesterol: 55mg
- Sodium: 150mg

Servings

- **4 servings**

Cooking Time

- **45 minutes**

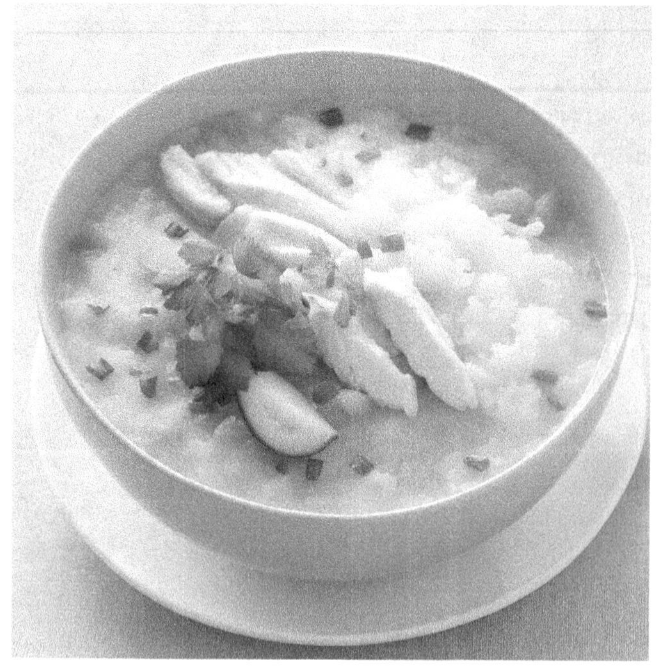

22. Turkey Spinach Wraps

Ingredients

- 1 pound cooked turkey breast, sliced
- 4 large whole wheat tortillas
- 2 cups fresh spinach leaves
- 1/2 cup plain Greek yogurt
- 1 tablespoon lemon juice
- 1/4 teaspoon ground black pepper
- 1/2 cup shredded carrots

Instructions

1. In a small bowl, mix the Greek yogurt, lemon juice, and ground black pepper.
2. Lay out the tortillas and spread a thin layer of the yogurt mixture on each one.
3. Top each tortilla with sliced turkey breast, fresh spinach leaves, and shredded carrots.
4. Roll up the tortillas tightly and slice in half before serving.

Nutrition Information (Per Serving)

- Calories: 320
- Protein: 28g
- Carbohydrates: 32g
- Dietary Fiber: 6g
- Sugars: 4g
- Fat: 10g
- Saturated Fat: 2g
- Cholesterol: 60mg
- Sodium: 300mg

Servings

- **4 servings**

Cooking Time

- **10 minutes**

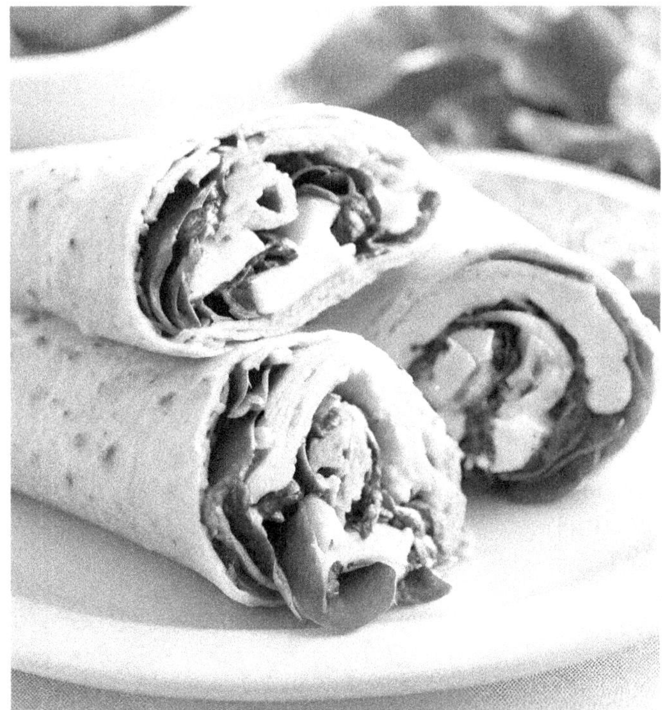

23. Chicken Quinoa Salad

Ingredients

- 1 pound boneless, skinless chicken breasts, cooked and diced
- 1 cup quinoa, rinsed
- 2 cups low-sodium chicken broth
- 1 cup diced cucumber
- 1 cup halved cherry tomatoes
- 1/4 cup chopped fresh parsley
- 2 tablespoons olive oil
- 1 tablespoon lemon juice
- 1/4 teaspoon ground black pepper

Instructions

1. In a medium saucepan, bring the chicken broth to a boil. Add the quinoa, reduce the heat to low, cover, and simmer for 15 minutes, or until the liquid is absorbed and the quinoa is tender.
2. In a large bowl, combine the cooked quinoa, diced chicken, cucumber, cherry tomatoes, and chopped parsley.
3. In a small bowl, whisk together the olive oil, lemon juice, and ground black pepper.
4. Pour the dressing over the salad and toss to combine.
5. Serve chilled or at room temperature.

Nutrition Information (Per Serving)

- Calories: 320
- Protein: 30g
- Carbohydrates: 28g
- Dietary Fiber: 5g
- Sugars: 4g
- Fat: 12g
- Saturated Fat: 2g
- Cholesterol: 60mg
- Sodium: 200mg

Servings

- **4 servings**

Cooking Time

- **20 minutes**

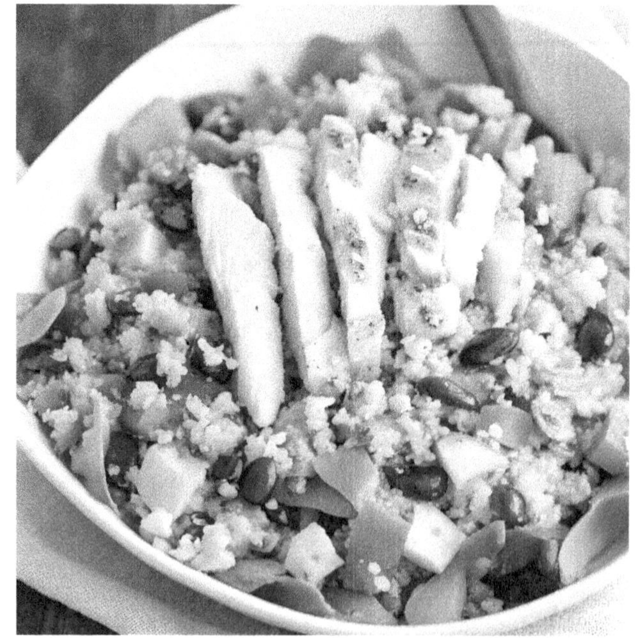

24. Chicken Muffins

Ingredients

- 1 pound ground chicken
- 1 cup grated zucchini
- 1/2 cup rolled oats
- 1 large egg, beaten
- 1/4 cup plain Greek yogurt
- 1 teaspoon dried thyme
- 1/4 teaspoon ground black pepper
- 2 tablespoons olive oil

Instructions

1. Preheat the oven to 375°F (190°C) and grease a muffin tin.
2. In a large bowl, combine the ground chicken, grated zucchini, rolled oats, beaten egg, Greek yogurt, dried thyme, and ground black pepper. Mix until well combined.
3. Divide the mixture evenly among the muffin cups.
4. Bake for 20-25 minutes, or until the muffins are cooked through and golden brown.
5. Let cool slightly before serving.

Nutrition Information (Per Serving)

- Calories: 180
- Protein: 25g
- Carbohydrates: 8g
- Dietary Fiber: 2g
- Sugars: 1g
- Fat: 7g
- Saturated Fat: 1.5g
- Cholesterol: 75mg
- Sodium: 90mg

Servings

- **4 servings**

Cooking Time

- **25 minutes**

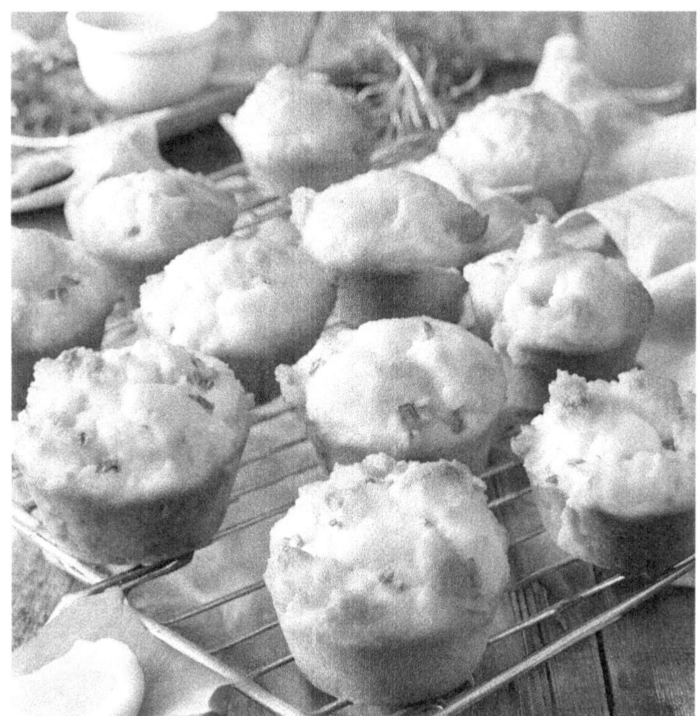

25. Turkey Stew with Vegetables

Ingredients

- 1 pound turkey breast, cubed
- 2 large carrots, diced
- 2 celery stalks, diced
- 1 cup diced potatoes
- 4 cups low-sodium chicken broth
- 1/2 cup unsweetened almond milk
- 2 tablespoons olive oil
- 1 teaspoon dried thyme
- 1/4 teaspoon ground black pepper

Instructions

1. In a large pot, heat the olive oil over medium heat.
2. Add the cubed turkey and cook for 5-7 minutes, until browned and cooked through. Remove from the pot and set aside.
3. In the same pot, add the diced carrots, celery, and potatoes. Cook for 5-7 minutes, stirring occasionally.
4. Add the chicken broth, dried thyme, and ground black pepper. Bring to a boil, then reduce the heat and simmer for 20 minutes, until the vegetables are tender.
5. Stir in the almond milk and return the turkey to the pot. Cook for an additional 5 minutes.
6. Serve hot.

Nutrition Information (Per Serving)

- Calories: 280
- Protein: 30g
- Carbohydrates: 18g
- Dietary Fiber: 4g
- Sugars: 4g
- Fat: 10g
- Saturated Fat: 1.5g
- Cholesterol: 65mg
- Sodium: 160mg

Servings

- **4 servings**

Cooking Time

- **40 minutes**

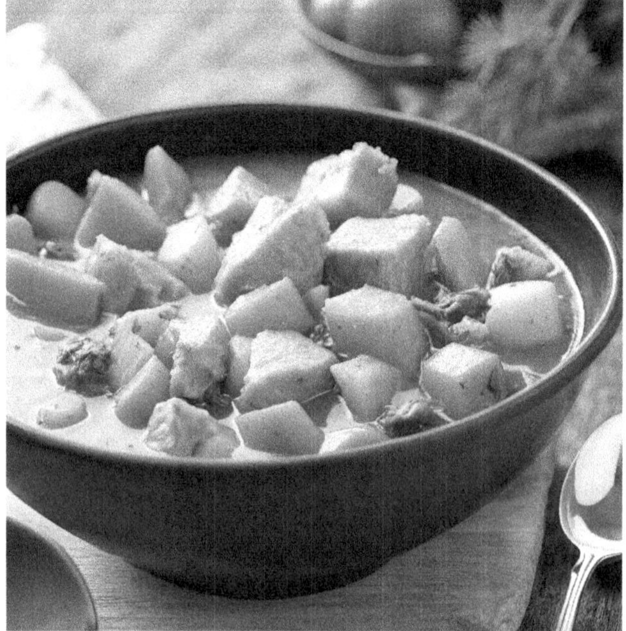

26. Chicken and Pear Bake

Ingredients

- 1 pound boneless, skinless chicken breasts, sliced
- 2 large pears, cored and sliced
- 1 cup baby spinach leaves
- 1/4 cup chopped walnuts
- 2 tablespoons olive oil
- 1 tablespoon lemon juice
- 1/4 teaspoon ground black pepper

Instructions

1. Preheat the oven to 375°F (190°C) and grease a baking dish.
2. In a small bowl, whisk together the olive oil, lemon juice, and ground black pepper.
3. Arrange the sliced chicken, pears, and spinach in the baking dish.
4. Drizzle with the olive oil mixture and sprinkle with chopped walnuts.
5. Bake for 25-30 minutes, or until the chicken is cooked through and the pears are tender.
6. Serve warm.

Nutrition Information (Per Serving)

- Calories: 290
- Protein: 28g
- Carbohydrates: 18g
- Dietary Fiber: 4g
- Sugars: 10g
- Fat: 12g
- Saturated Fat: 2g
- Cholesterol: 65mg
- Sodium: 140mg

Servings

- **4 servings**

Cooking Time

- **30 minutes**

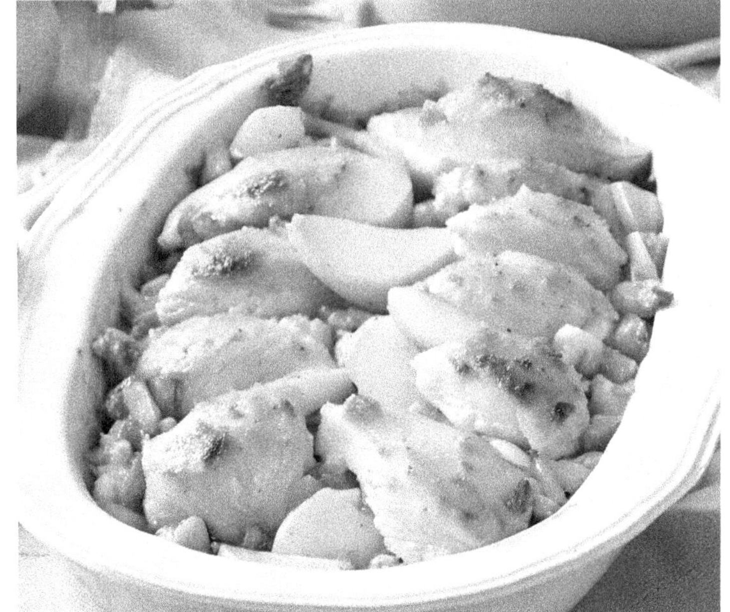

27. Chicken Noodle Casserole

Ingredients

- 1 pound boneless, skinless chicken breasts, diced
- 8 ounces whole wheat egg noodles
- 1 cup diced carrots
- 1 cup frozen peas
- 1 cup unsweetened almond milk
- 1/2 cup low-sodium chicken broth
- 1/4 cup grated Parmesan cheese
- 2 tablespoons olive oil
- 1 teaspoon dried basil
- 1/4 teaspoon ground black pepper

Instructions

1. Preheat the oven to 375°F (190°C) and grease a baking dish.
2. Cook the egg noodles according to package instructions. Drain and set aside.
3. In a large skillet, heat the olive oil over medium heat.
4. Add the diced chicken and cook for 5-7 minutes, until browned and cooked through. Remove from the skillet and set aside.
5. In the same skillet, add the diced carrots and cook for 5 minutes, until slightly tender.
6. Stir in the almond milk, chicken broth, dried basil, and ground black pepper. Bring to a simmer.
7. Add the cooked chicken, frozen peas, and cooked egg noodles to the skillet. Stir to combine.
8. Transfer the mixture to the prepared baking dish and sprinkle with grated Parmesan cheese.
9. Bake for 20-25 minutes, until the top is golden brown and the casserole is heated through.
10. Serve warm.

Nutrition Information (Per Serving)

- Calories: 320
- Protein: 30g
- Carbohydrates: 35g
- Dietary Fiber: 5g
- Sugars: 4g
- Fat: 10g
- Saturated Fat: 2g
- Cholesterol: 65mg
- Sodium: 200mg

Servings

- **4 servings**

Cooking Time

- **30 minutes**

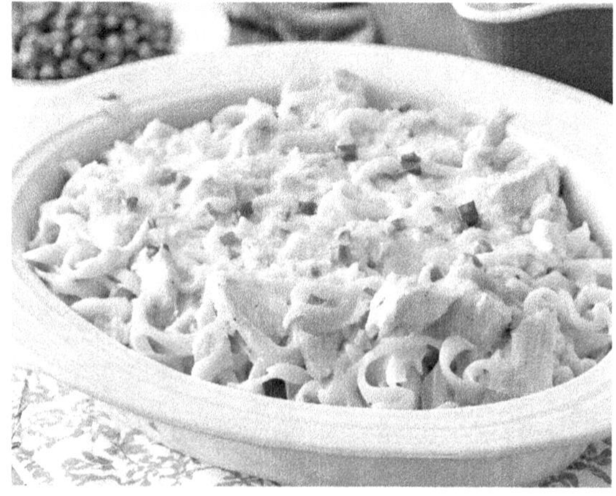

28. Roast Turkey Breast

Ingredients

- 1 whole turkey breast (about 4 pounds)
- 2 tablespoons olive oil
- 1 tablespoon dried rosemary
- 1 tablespoon dried thyme
- 1/4 teaspoon ground black pepper

Instructions

1. Preheat the oven to 350°F (175°C) and line a roasting pan with parchment paper.
2. In a small bowl, mix the olive oil, dried rosemary, dried thyme, and ground black pepper.
3. Rub the mixture over the turkey breast.
4. Place the turkey breast in the prepared roasting pan.
5. Roast for 1 hour and 30 minutes, or until the internal temperature reaches 165°F (75°C).
6. Let the turkey rest for 10 minutes before slicing.
7. Serve warm.

Nutrition Information (Per Serving)

- Calories: 280
- Protein: 35g
- Carbohydrates: 1g
- Dietary Fiber: 0g
- Sugars: 0g
- Fat: 15g
- Saturated Fat: 3g
- Cholesterol: 95mg
- Sodium: 120mg

Servings

- **8 servings**

Cooking Time

- **1 hour 40 minutes**

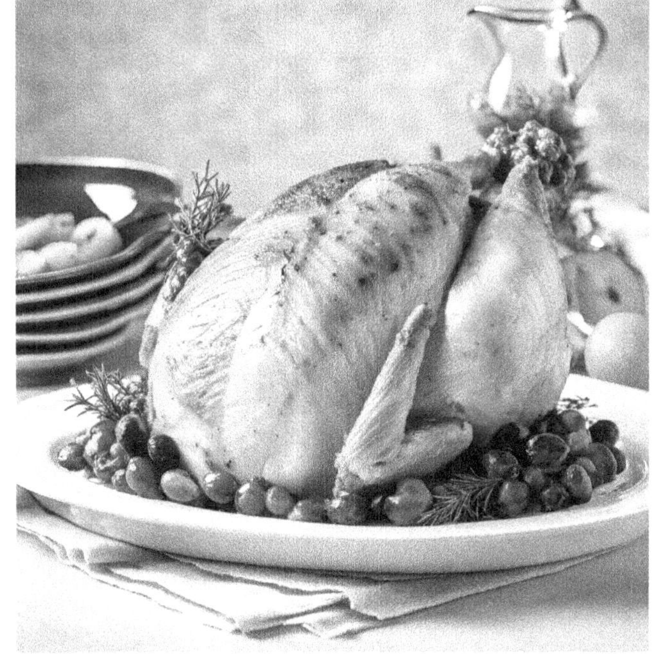

Desserts

1. Banana Pudding
Ingredients
- 3 ripe bananas, sliced
- 2 cups unsweetened almond milk
- 1/4 cup cornstarch
- 1/3 cup honey
- 1 teaspoon vanilla extract
- 1/4 teaspoon ground cinnamon

Instructions
1. In a medium saucepan, combine the almond milk and cornstarch. Whisk until smooth.
2. Add the honey and cook over medium heat, stirring constantly, until the mixture thickens and begins to boil.
3. Remove from heat and stir in the vanilla extract and ground cinnamon.
4. In a serving dish, layer the banana slices and pour the pudding mixture over them.
5. Refrigerate for at least 2 hours before serving.

Nutrition Information (Per Serving)
- Calories: 150
- Protein: 2g
- Carbohydrates: 35g
- Dietary Fiber: 2g
- Sugars: 25g
- Fat: 1g
- Saturated Fat: 0g
- Cholesterol: 0mg
- Sodium: 50mg

Servings
- **4 servings**

Cooking Time
- **10 minutes prep, 2 hours chilling**

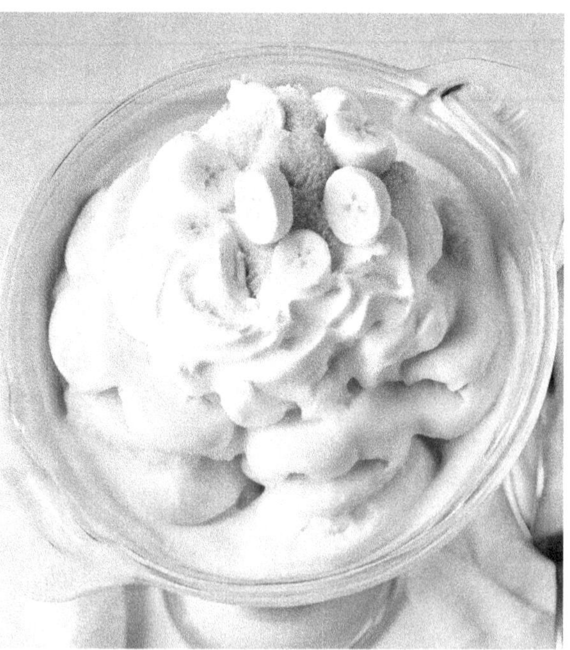

2. Oatmeal Cookies
Ingredients
- 1 cup rolled oats
- 1/2 cup whole wheat flour
- 1/2 teaspoon baking soda
- 1/4 cup honey
- 1/4 cup unsweetened applesauce
- 1/4 cup olive oil
- 1 teaspoon vanilla extract
- 1/2 teaspoon ground cinnamon

Instructions
1. Preheat the oven to 350°F (175°C) and line a baking sheet with parchment paper.
2. In a large bowl, combine the rolled oats, whole wheat flour, and baking soda.
3. In another bowl, mix the honey, applesauce, olive oil, vanilla extract, and ground cinnamon.
4. Add the wet ingredients to the dry ingredients and mix until combined.
5. Drop spoonfuls of the dough onto the prepared baking sheet.
6. Bake for 10-12 minutes, or until the cookies are golden brown.
7. Let cool on the baking sheet for 5 minutes before transferring to a wire rack to cool completely.

Nutrition Information (Per Serving)
- Calories: 90
- Protein: 1g
- Carbohydrates: 15g
- Dietary Fiber: 2g
- Sugars: 8g
- Fat: 3g
- Saturated Fat: 0.5g
- Cholesterol: 0mg
- Sodium: 50mg

Servings
- **12 cookies**

Cooking Time
- **15 minutes**

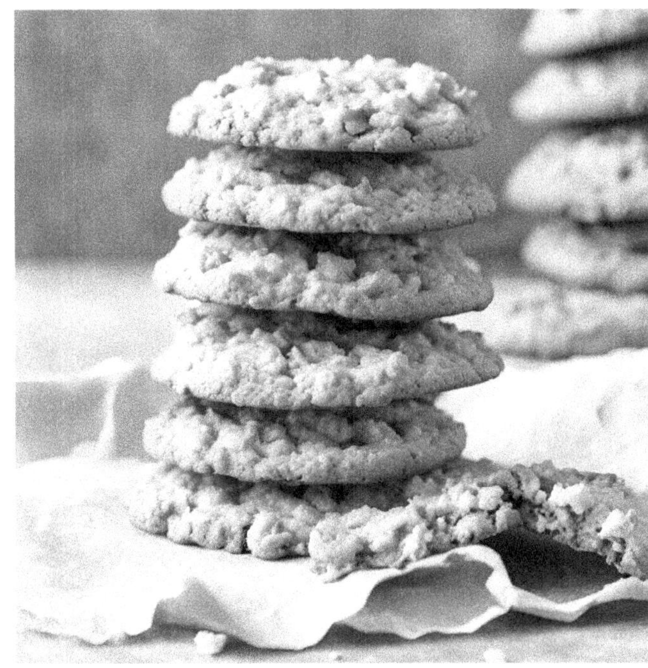

3. Pumpkin Pie

Ingredients

- 1 pre-made whole wheat pie crust
- 1 can (15 ounces) pumpkin puree
- 1 cup unsweetened almond milk
- 2/3 cup honey
- 3 large eggs
- 1 teaspoon ground cinnamon
- 1/2 teaspoon ground ginger
- 1/4 teaspoon ground nutmeg

Instructions

1. Preheat the oven to 375°F (190°C).
2. In a large bowl, whisk together the pumpkin puree, almond milk, honey, eggs, ground cinnamon, ground ginger, and ground nutmeg until smooth.
3. Pour the mixture into the pie crust.
4. Bake for 50-55 minutes, or until a knife inserted into the center comes out clean.
5. Let the pie cool completely before serving.

Nutrition Information (Per Serving)

- Calories: 200
- Protein: 4g
- Carbohydrates: 35g
- Dietary Fiber: 3g
- Sugars: 20g
- Fat: 6g
- Saturated Fat: 1.5g
- Cholesterol: 60mg
- Sodium: 150mg

Servings

- **8 servings**

Cooking Time

- **1 hour**

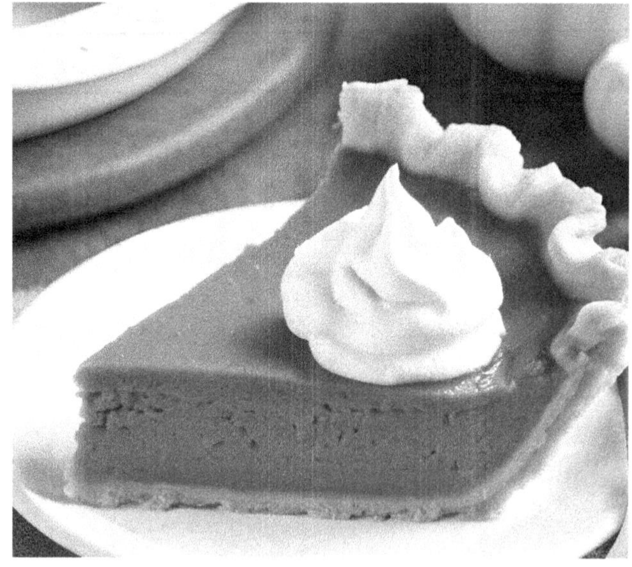

4. Apple Compote

Ingredients

- 4 large apples, peeled, cored, and diced
- 1/2 cup water
- 1/4 cup honey
- 1 teaspoon ground cinnamon
- 1/4 teaspoon ground ginger

Instructions

1. In a large saucepan, combine the diced apples, water, honey, ground cinnamon, and ground ginger.
2. Cook over medium heat, stirring occasionally, until the apples are soft and the mixture has thickened, about 15-20 minutes.
3. Serve warm or chilled.

Nutrition Information (Per Serving)

- Calories: 120
- Protein: 0g
- Carbohydrates: 31g
- Dietary Fiber: 4g
- Sugars: 25g
- Fat: 0g
- Saturated Fat: 0g
- Cholesterol: 0mg
- Sodium: 10mg

Servings

- **4 servings**

Cooking Time

- **20 minutes**

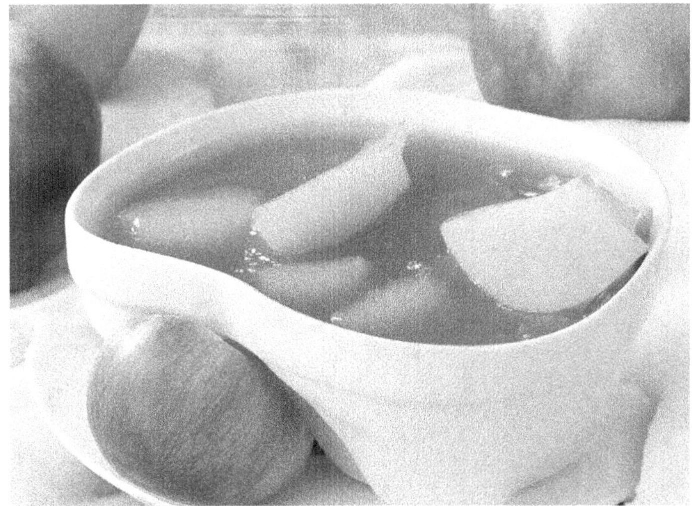

5. Blueberry Yogurt Parfait

Ingredients

- 2 cups plain Greek yogurt
- 1 cup fresh blueberries
- 1/4 cup honey
- 1/2 cup granola (low-sugar)

Instructions

1. In a bowl, mix the Greek yogurt and honey until well combined.
2. In serving glasses or bowls, layer the yogurt mixture, fresh blueberries, and granola.
3. Repeat the layers until all ingredients are used, finishing with a layer of granola on top.
4. Serve immediately or refrigerate until ready to serve.

Nutrition Information (Per Serving)

- Calories: 180
- Protein: 10g
- Carbohydrates: 28g
- Dietary Fiber: 2g
- Sugars: 20g
- Fat: 4g
- Saturated Fat: 1g
- Cholesterol: 10mg
- Sodium: 50mg

Servings

- **4 servings**

Cooking Time

- **10 minutes**

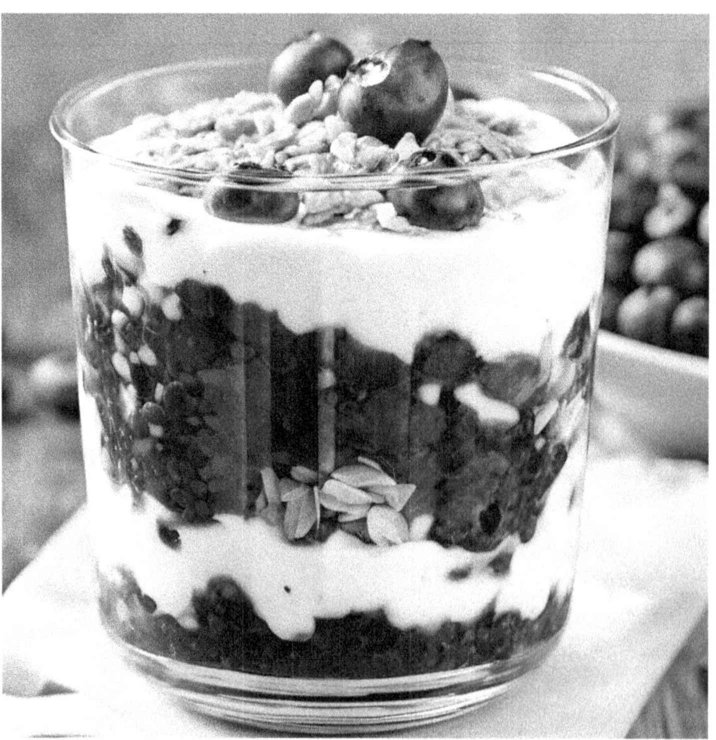

6. Vanilla Custard

Ingredients

- 2 cups unsweetened almond milk
- 4 large egg yolks
- 1/4 cup honey
- 2 tablespoons cornstarch
- 1 teaspoon vanilla extract
- 1/4 teaspoon ground cinnamon

Instructions

1. In a medium saucepan, heat the almond milk over medium heat until it begins to simmer. Do not let it boil.
2. In a bowl, whisk together the egg yolks, honey, and cornstarch until smooth.
3. Gradually whisk the hot almond milk into the egg mixture.
4. Return the mixture to the saucepan and cook over medium heat, stirring constantly, until the custard thickens and coats the back of a spoon.
5. Remove from heat and stir in the vanilla extract and ground cinnamon.
6. Pour the custard into serving dishes and refrigerate for at least 2 hours before serving.

Nutrition Information (Per Serving)

- Calories: 140
- Protein: 4g
- Carbohydrates: 22g
- Dietary Fiber: 0g
- Sugars: 20g
- Fat: 4g
- Saturated Fat: 1g
- Cholesterol: 120mg
- Sodium: 45mg

Servings

- **4 servings**

Cooking Time

- **20 minutes prep, 2 hours chilling**

7. Maple Syrup Pancakes

Ingredients

- 1 cup whole wheat flour
- 1 tablespoon baking powder
- 1 cup unsweetened almond milk
- 1 large egg
- 2 tablespoons olive oil
- 1/4 cup pure maple syrup

Instructions

1. In a large bowl, whisk together the whole wheat flour and baking powder.
2. In another bowl, mix the almond milk, egg, and olive oil.
3. Add the wet ingredients to the dry ingredients and stir until just combined.
4. Heat a non-stick skillet over medium heat and lightly grease with olive oil.
5. Pour 1/4 cup of batter onto the skillet for each pancake. Cook until bubbles form on the surface, then flip and cook until golden brown on the other side.
6. Serve the pancakes warm, drizzled with pure maple syrup.

Nutrition Information (Per Serving)

- Calories: 150
- Protein: 4g
- Carbohydrates: 26g
- Dietary Fiber: 3g
- Sugars: 8g
- Fat: 5g
- Saturated Fat: 1g
- Cholesterol: 35mg
- Sodium: 150mg

Servings

- **4 servings**

Cooking Time

- **20 minutes**

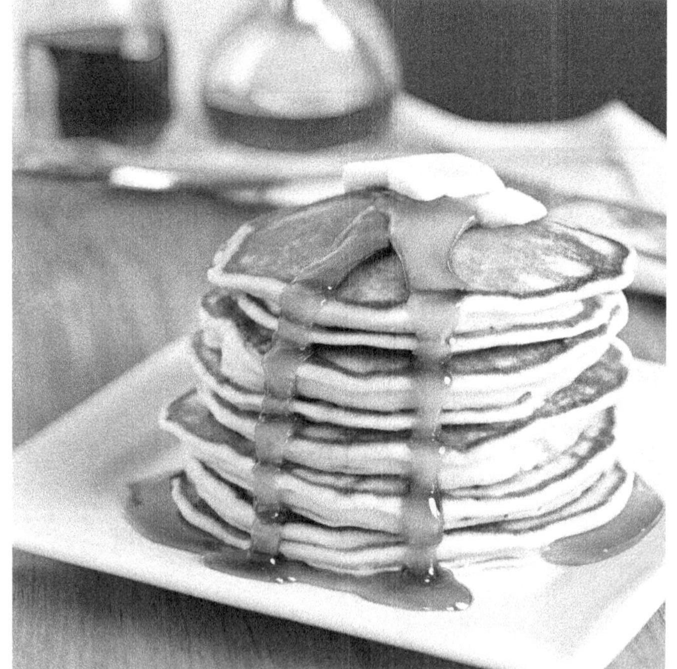

8. Sweet Potato Pie

Ingredients

- 1 pre-made whole wheat pie crust
- 2 cups mashed sweet potatoes
- 1 cup unsweetened almond milk
- 1/2 cup honey
- 2 large eggs
- 1 teaspoon ground cinnamon
- 1/2 teaspoon ground nutmeg
- 1/4 teaspoon ground ginger

Instructions

1. Preheat the oven to 375°F (190°C).
2. In a large bowl, whisk together the mashed sweet potatoes, almond milk, honey, eggs, ground cinnamon, ground nutmeg, and ground ginger until smooth.
3. Pour the mixture into the pie crust.
4. Bake for 45-50 minutes, or until the pie is set and a knife inserted into the center comes out clean.
5. Let the pie cool completely before serving.

Nutrition Information (Per Serving)

- Calories: 220
- Protein: 4g
- Carbohydrates: 38g
- Dietary Fiber: 4g
- Sugars: 18g
- Fat: 7g
- Saturated Fat: 1.5g
- Cholesterol: 55mg
- Sodium: 140mg

Servings

- **8 servings**

Cooking Time

- **50 minutes**

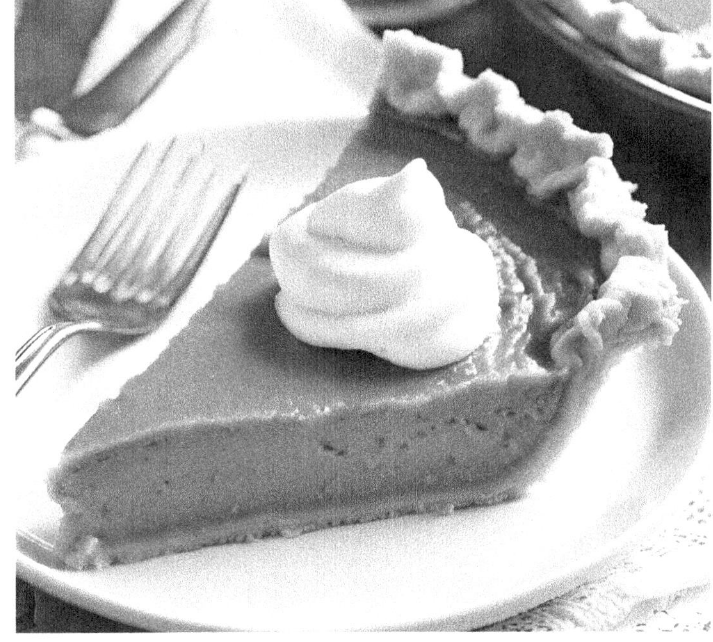

9. Banana Smoothie

Ingredients

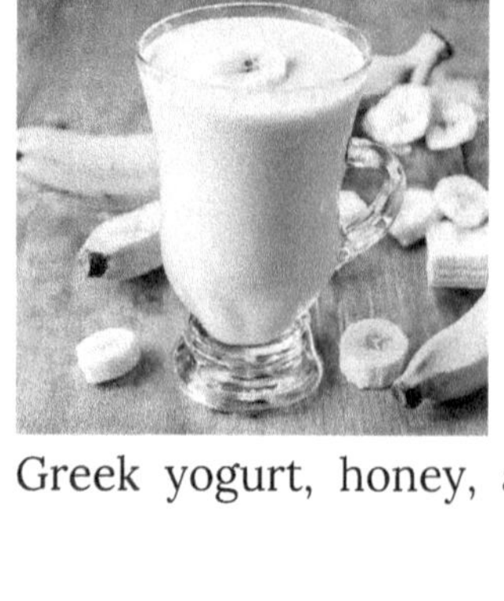

- 2 ripe bananas
- 1 cup unsweetened almond milk
- 1/2 cup plain Greek yogurt
- 1 tablespoon honey
- 1/2 teaspoon vanilla extract

Instructions

1. In a blender, combine the bananas, almond milk, Greek yogurt, honey, and vanilla extract.
2. Blend until smooth and creamy.
3. Pour into glasses and serve immediately.

Nutrition Information (Per Serving)

- Calories: 150   Protein: 4g Carbohydrates: 30g Dietary Fiber: 3g
- Sugars: 20g Fat: 2g Saturated Fat: 0.5g Cholesterol: 5mg Sodium: 45mg

Servings

- **2 servings**

Cooking Time

- **5 minutes**

10. Strawberry Shake

Ingredients

- 1 cup fresh strawberries, hulled and sliced
- 1 cup unsweetened almond milk
- 1/2 cup plain Greek yogurt
- 1 tablespoon honey
- 1/2 teaspoon vanilla extract

Instructions

1. In a blender, combine the strawberries, almond milk, Greek yogurt, honey, and vanilla extract.
2. Blend until smooth and creamy.
3. Pour into glasses and serve immediately.

Nutrition Information (Per Serving)

- Calories: 130   Protein: 5g Carbohydrates: 24g Dietary Fiber: 2g
- Sugars: 18g Fat: 2g Saturated Fat: 0.5g Cholesterol: 5mg
- Sodium: 40mg

Servings

- **2 servings**

Cooking Time

- **5 minutes**

10-WEEK MEAL PLAN

Week 1

Day 1
- Breakfast: Avocado and Egg Breakfast Cups
- Lunch: Chicken and Rice Porridge
- Dinner: Roasted Chicken with Root Vegetables
- Snack: Banana Pudding

Day 2
- Breakfast: Low Carb Breakfast Burritos
- Lunch: Turkey Spinach Wraps
- Dinner: Grilled Turkey Tenderloin
- Snack: Oatmeal Cookies

Day 3
- Breakfast: Air Fryer Omelet with Spinach and Cheese
- Lunch: Chicken Quinoa Salad
- Dinner: Turkey Stew with Vegetables
- Snack: Pear Nectar

Day 4
- Breakfast: Sausage and Cheese Stuffed Mushrooms
- Lunch: Chicken Muffins
- Dinner: Chicken Pilaf
- Snack: Vanilla Custard

Day 5
- Breakfast: Zucchini Hash Browns
- Lunch: Turkey and Carrot Patties
- Dinner: Herbed Turkey Steaks
- Snack: Papaya Smoothie

Day 6
- Breakfast: Low Carb Pancakes
- Lunch: Turkey Bolognese
- Dinner: Turkey Pot Pie
- Snack: Fig Smoothie

Day 7
- Breakfast: Air Fryer Bacon and Eggs
- Lunch: Chicken Noodle Casserole
- Dinner: Roast Turkey Breast
- Snack: Maple Syrup Pancakes

Week 2

Day 1
- Breakfast: Keto Breakfast Sandwich
- Lunch: Chicken Sweet Potato Hash
- Dinner: Chicken with Parsley Pesto
- Snack: Blueberry Yogurt Parfait

Day 2
- Breakfast: Cauliflower Breakfast Muffins
- Lunch: Stuffed Chicken Breasts
- Dinner: Chicken Minestrone Soup
- Snack: Lemon Balm Tea

Day 3
- Breakfast: Low Carb French Toast Sticks
- Lunch: Turkey Vegetable Loaf
- Dinner: Turkey Cranberry Wraps
- Snack: Apple Compote

Day 4
- Breakfast: Air Fryer Cinnamon Rolls
- Lunch: Grilled Chicken with Avocado Salad
- Dinner: Turkey and Apple Stew
- Snack: Strawberry Shake

Day 5
- Breakfast: Cheesy Egg Bites
- Lunch: Chicken with Mushrooms
- Dinner: Chicken and Pear Bake
- Snack: Oat Milk Smoothie

Day 6
- Breakfast: Broccoli and Cheese Breakfast Casserole
- Lunch: Turkey Oatmeal Meatballs
- Dinner: Sweet Potato Pie
- Snack: Berry Compote

Day 7
- Breakfast: Low Carb Blueberry Muffins
- Lunch: Chicken and Barley Stew
- Dinner: Creamy Chicken Alfredo
- Snack: Pineapple Coconut Smoothie

Week 3

Day 1
- Breakfast: Spinach and Feta Stuffed Peppers
- Lunch: Turkey Spinach Wraps
- Dinner: Grilled Turkey Tenderloin
- Snack: Vanilla Custard

Day 2

- Breakfast: Almond Flour Waffles
- Lunch: Chicken Quinoa Salad
- Dinner: Roasted Chicken with Root Vegetables
- Snack: Pear Nectar

Day 3

- Breakfast: Keto Bagels
- Lunch: Turkey Stew with Vegetables
- Dinner: Turkey Pot Pie
- Snack: Oatmeal Cookies

Day 4

- Breakfast: Air Fryer Chia Pudding
- Lunch: Chicken Pilaf
- Dinner: Turkey and Apple Stew
- Snack: Maple Syrup Pancakes

Day 5

- Breakfast: Eggplant Bacon
- Lunch: Chicken Muffins
- Dinner: Herbed Turkey Steaks
- Snack: Fig Smoothie

Day 6

- Breakfast: Air Fryer Breakfast Sausage Patties
- Lunch: Turkey and Carrot Patties
- Dinner: Chicken Noodle Casserole
- Snack: Lemon Balm Tea

Day 7

- Breakfast: Zucchini Hash Browns
- Lunch: Chicken Sweet Potato Hash
- Dinner: Roast Turkey Breast
- Snack: Papaya Smoothie

Week 4

Day 1

- Breakfast: Air Fryer Omelet with Spinach and Cheese
- Lunch: Turkey Spinach Wraps
- Dinner: Chicken with Parsley Pesto
- Snack: Blueberry Yogurt Parfait

Day 2

- Breakfast: Low Carb Pancakes
- Lunch: Grilled Chicken with Avocado Salad
- Dinner: Chicken and Pear Bake
- Snack: Strawberry Shake

Day 3
- Breakfast: Air Fryer Bacon and Eggs
- Lunch: Chicken with Mushrooms
- Dinner: Creamy Chicken Alfredo
- Snack: Berry Compote

Day 4
- Breakfast: Keto Breakfast Sandwich
- Lunch: Stuffed Chicken Breasts
- Dinner: Chicken Minestrone Soup
- Snack: Pineapple Coconut Smoothie

Day 5
- Breakfast: Cauliflower Breakfast Muffins
- Lunch: Turkey Oatmeal Meatballs
- Dinner: Turkey Cranberry Wraps
- Snack: Apple Compote

Day 6
- Breakfast: Low Carb French Toast Sticks
- Lunch: Turkey Vegetable Loaf
- Dinner: Turkey Bolognese
- Snack: Oat Milk Smoothie

Day 7
- Breakfast: Cheesy Egg Bites
- Lunch: Chicken and Barley Stew
- Dinner: Turkey Stew with Vegetables
- Snack: Vanilla Custard

Week 5

Day 1
- Breakfast: Broccoli and Cheese Breakfast Casserole
- Lunch: Turkey and Carrot Patties
- Dinner: Grilled Turkey Tenderloin
- Snack: Pear Nectar

Day 2
- Breakfast: Low Carb Blueberry Muffins
- Lunch: Chicken Sweet Potato Hash
- Dinner: Chicken Noodle Casserole
- Snack: Maple Syrup Pancakes

Day 3
- Breakfast: Spinach and Feta Stuffed Peppers
- Lunch: Turkey Spinach Wraps
- Dinner: Turkey and Apple Stew
- Snack: Fig Smoothie

Day 4

- Breakfast: Almond Flour Waffles
- Lunch: Chicken Muffins
- Dinner: Herbed Turkey Steaks
- Snack: Lemon Balm Tea

Day 5

- Breakfast: Keto Bagels
- Lunch: Chicken Pilaf
- Dinner: Chicken with Parsley Pesto
- Snack: Blueberry Yogurt Parfait

Day 6

- Breakfast: Air Fryer Chia Pudding
- Lunch: Grilled Chicken with Avocado Salad
- Dinner: Chicken and Pear Bake
- Snack: Pineapple Coconut Smoothie

Day 7

- Breakfast: Eggplant Bacon
- Lunch: Chicken Quinoa Salad
- Dinner: Roast Turkey Breast
- Snack: Strawberry Shake

Week 6

Day 1

- Breakfast: Low Carb Breakfast Burritos
- Lunch: Chicken Sweet Potato Hash
- Dinner: Turkey and Apple Stew
- Snack: Pear Nectar

Day 2

- Breakfast: Air Fryer Omelet with Spinach and Cheese
- Lunch: Chicken Quinoa Salad
- Dinner: Chicken and Barley Stew
- Snack: Oat Milk Smoothie

Day 3

- Breakfast: Sausage and Cheese Stuffed Mushrooms
- Lunch: Turkey Cranberry Wraps
- Dinner: Chicken Noodle Casserole
- Snack: Berry Compote

Day 4

- Breakfast: Zucchini Hash Browns
- Lunch: Stuffed Chicken Breasts
- Dinner: Turkey Stew with Vegetables
- Snack: Pineapple Coconut Smoothie

Day 5

- Breakfast: Low Carb Pancakes
- Lunch: Chicken with Mushrooms
- Dinner: Turkey Pot Pie
- Snack: Vanilla Custard

Day 6

- Breakfast: Air Fryer Bacon and Eggs
- Lunch: Grilled Turkey Tenderloin
- Dinner: Chicken with Parsley Pesto
- Snack: Fig Smoothie

Day 7

- Breakfast: Keto Breakfast Sandwich
- Lunch: Turkey Vegetable Loaf
- Dinner: Chicken Pilaf
- Snack: Apple Compote

Week 7

Day 1

- Breakfast: Cauliflower Breakfast Muffins
- Lunch: Chicken and Rice Porridge
- Dinner: Herbed Turkey Steaks
- Snack: Papaya Smoothie

Day 2

- Breakfast: Low Carb French Toast Sticks
- Lunch: Turkey and Carrot Patties
- Dinner: Chicken and Pear Bake
- Snack: Maple Syrup Pancakes

Day 3

- Breakfast: Air Fryer Cinnamon Rolls
- Lunch: Chicken Muffins
- Dinner: Chicken Minestrone Soup
- Snack: Lemon Balm Tea

Day 4

- Breakfast: Cheesy Egg Bites
- Lunch: Chicken Sweet Potato Hash
- Dinner: Turkey and Apple Stew
- Snack: Blueberry Yogurt Parfait

Day 5

- Breakfast: Broccoli and Cheese Breakfast Casserole
- Lunch: Chicken Quinoa Salad
- Dinner: Turkey Cranberry Wraps
- Snack: Oat Milk Smoothie

Day 6
- Breakfast: Low Carb Blueberry Muffins
- Lunch: Chicken and Barley Stew
- Dinner: Turkey Stew with Vegetables
- Snack: Strawberry Shake

Day 7
- Breakfast: Spinach and Feta Stuffed Peppers
- Lunch: Stuffed Chicken Breasts
- Dinner: Chicken Noodle Casserole
- Snack: Pear Nectar

Week 8

Day 1
- Breakfast: Almond Flour Waffles
- Lunch: Grilled Turkey Tenderloin
- Dinner: Chicken with Parsley Pesto
- Snack: Berry Compote

Day 2
- Breakfast: Keto Bagels
- Lunch: Chicken with Mushrooms
- Dinner: Turkey Pot Pie
- Snack: Pineapple Coconut Smoothie

Day 3
- Breakfast: Air Fryer Chia Pudding
- Lunch: Chicken and Rice Porridge
- Dinner: Chicken Pilaf
- Snack: Vanilla Custard

Day 4
- Breakfast: Eggplant Bacon
- Lunch: Turkey Vegetable Loaf
- Dinner: Herbed Turkey Steaks
- Snack: Fig Smoothie

Day 5
- Breakfast: Air Fryer Breakfast Sausage Patties
- Lunch: Chicken Muffins
- Dinner: Chicken Minestrone Soup
- Snack: Maple Syrup Pancakes

Day 6
- Breakfast: Zucchini Hash Browns
- Lunch: Turkey and Carrot Patties
- Dinner: Chicken and Pear Bake
- Snack: Apple Compote

Day 7
- Breakfast: Air Fryer Omelet with Spinach and Cheese
- Lunch: Chicken Quinoa Salad
- Dinner: Turkey Cranberry Wraps
- Snack: Lemon Balm Tea

Week 9

Day 1
- Breakfast: Low Carb Breakfast Burritos
- Lunch: Chicken Sweet Potato Hash
- Dinner: Turkey and Apple Stew
- Snack: Blueberry Yogurt Parfait

Day 2
- Breakfast: Sausage and Cheese Stuffed Mushrooms
- Lunch: Stuffed Chicken Breasts
- Dinner: Chicken Noodle Casserole
- Snack: Pear Nectar

Day 3
- Breakfast: Low Carb Pancakes
- Lunch: Turkey Vegetable Loaf
- Dinner: Chicken Pilaf
- Snack: Berry Compote

Day 4
- Breakfast: Air Fryer Bacon and Eggs
- Lunch: Turkey and Carrot Patties
- Dinner: Chicken and Rice Porridge
- Snack: Papaya Smoothie

Day 5
- Breakfast: Keto Breakfast Sandwich
- Lunch: Chicken with Mushrooms
- Dinner: Turkey Pot Pie
- Snack: Oat Milk Smoothie

Day 6
- Breakfast: Cauliflower Breakfast Muffins
- Lunch: Grilled Turkey Tenderloin
- Dinner: Chicken with Parsley Pesto
- Snack: Pineapple Coconut Smoothie

Day 7
- Breakfast: Low Carb French Toast Sticks
- Lunch: Chicken Muffins
- Dinner: Turkey Stew with Vegetables
- Snack: Strawberry Shake

Week 10

Day 1
- Breakfast: Air Fryer Cinnamon Rolls
- Lunch: Chicken Quinoa Salad
- Dinner: Chicken Minestrone Soup
- Snack: Vanilla Custard

Day 2
- Breakfast: Cheesy Egg Bites
- Lunch: Turkey Cranberry Wraps
- Dinner: Chicken Pilaf
- Snack: Maple Syrup Pancakes

Day 3
- Breakfast: Broccoli and Cheese Breakfast Casserole
- Lunch: Stuffed Chicken Breasts
- Dinner: Chicken Noodle Casserole
- Snack: Fig Smoothie

Day 4
- Breakfast: Low Carb Blueberry Muffins
- Lunch: Chicken Sweet Potato Hash
- Dinner: Turkey and Apple Stew
- Snack: Pear Nectar

Day 5
- Breakfast: Spinach and Feta Stuffed Peppers
- Lunch: Turkey Vegetable Loaf
- Dinner: Chicken and Barley Stew
- Snack: Berry Compote

Day 6
- Breakfast: Almond Flour Waffles
- Lunch: Turkey and Carrot Patties
- Dinner: Herbed Turkey Steaks
- Snack: Pineapple Coconut Smoothie

Day 7
- Breakfast: Keto Bagels
- Lunch: Chicken Muffins
- Dinner: Turkey Pot Pie
- Snack: Vanilla Custard

WEEKLY MEAL PLANNER + WORKBOOK

	BREAKFAST	LUNCH	DINNER	SNACKS
MONDAY				
TUESDAY				
WEDNESDAY				
THURSDAY				
FRIDAY				
SATURDAY				
SUNDAY				

Reflect on your current symptoms. How are they impacting your daily life and eating habits?

WEEKLY MEAL PLANNER + WORKBOOK

	BREAKFAST	LUNCH	DINNER	SNACKS
MONDAY				
TUESDAY				
WEDNESDAY				
THURSDAY				
FRIDAY				
SATURDAY				
SUNDAY				

List three foods or beverages that you suspect might trigger discomfort or worsen your symptoms. How do you plan to avoid them?

WEEKLY MEAL PLANNER + WORKBOOK

	BREAKFAST	LUNCH	DINNER	SNACKS
MONDAY				
TUESDAY				
WEDNESDAY				
THURSDAY				
FRIDAY				
SATURDAY				
SUNDAY				

Consider your typical meal patterns before your ulcer diagnosis. What changes do you anticipate making to align with the gastric ulcer diet?

....

....

....

....

....

WEEKLY MEAL PLANNER + WORKBOOK

	BREAKFAST	LUNCH	DINNER	SNACKS
MONDAY				
TUESDAY				
WEDNESDAY				
THURSDAY				
FRIDAY				
SATURDAY				
SUNDAY				

Reflect on your hydration habits. How do you plan to ensure you're drinking enough fluids while managing ulcer symptoms?

....

....

....

....

....

WEEKLY MEAL PLANNER + WORKBOOK

	BREAKFAST	LUNCH	DINNER	SNACKS
MONDAY				
TUESDAY				
WEDNESDAY				
THURSDAY				
FRIDAY				
SATURDAY				
SUNDAY				

Identify any dietary habits or preferences that you believe might need to change to support your healing. Why are these changes important?

WEEKLY MEAL PLANNER + WORKBOOK

	BREAKFAST	LUNCH	DINNER	SNACKS
MONDAY				
TUESDAY				
WEDNESDAY				
THURSDAY				
FRIDAY				
SATURDAY				
SUNDAY				

What are your main concerns or challenges about starting the gastric ulcer diet? How do you plan to address these concerns?

WEEKLY MEAL PLANNER + WORKBOOK

	BREAKFAST	LUNCH	DINNER	SNACKS
MONDAY				
TUESDAY				
WEDNESDAY				
THURSDAY				
FRIDAY				
SATURDAY				
SUNDAY				

List three new foods or ingredients recommended for the gastric ulcer diet that you're willing to incorporate into your meals. What benefits do you expect from including these items?

WEEKLY MEAL PLANNER + WORKBOOK

	BREAKFAST	LUNCH	DINNER	SNACKS
MONDAY				
TUESDAY				
WEDNESDAY				
THURSDAY				
FRIDAY				
SATURDAY				
SUNDAY				

How do you plan to navigate social situations or dining out while adhering to the gastric ulcer diet?

WEEKLY MEAL PLANNER + WORKBOOK

	BREAKFAST	LUNCH	DINNER	SNACKS
MONDAY				
TUESDAY				
WEDNESDAY				
THURSDAY				
FRIDAY				
SATURDAY				
SUNDAY				

Consider your support system. How can family members or friends assist you in maintaining the gastric ulcer diet?

WEEKLY MEAL PLANNER + WORKBOOK

	BREAKFAST	LUNCH	DINNER	SNACKS
MONDAY				
TUESDAY				
WEDNESDAY				
THURSDAY				
FRIDAY				
SATURDAY				
SUNDAY				

What strategies will you use to track your food intake and monitor how your body responds to different foods on the gastric ulcer diet?

WEEKLY MEAL PLANNER + WORKBOOK

	BREAKFAST	LUNCH	DINNER	SNACKS
MONDAY				
TUESDAY				
WEDNESDAY				
THURSDAY				
FRIDAY				
SATURDAY				
SUNDAY				

Think about your favorite meals and snacks before your ulcer diagnosis. How can you adapt these to fit within the guidelines of the gastric ulcer diet?

WEEKLY MEAL PLANNER + WORKBOOK

	BREAKFAST	LUNCH	DINNER	SNACKS
MONDAY				
TUESDAY				
WEDNESDAY				
THURSDAY				
FRIDAY				
SATURDAY				
SUNDAY				

Consider any medications you're currently taking. How do you plan to coordinate your diet with your medication schedule?

Scan the QR code below to get a surprise bonus!